CREATION OF CALM
A Cancer Survivor's Sketchbook Story

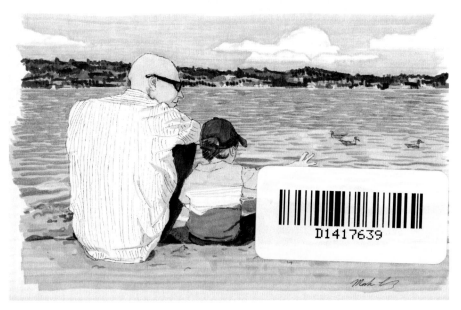

ILLUSTRATED & WRITTEN

BY Mark Fraley

Creation of Calm: A Cancer Survivor's Sketchbook Story
© 2014 by Mark Fraley

Published by Cladach Publishing
PO Box 336144 Greeley, CO 80633
www.cladach.com

Unless otherwise indicated, all Scripture quotations are taken from THE MES-
SAGE. Copyright © by Eugene H. Peterson 1993, 1994, 1995, 1996, 2000, 2001,
2002. Used by permission of Tyndale House Publishers, Inc.
Scripture quotation marked ISV is taken from the Holy Bible: International
Standard Version®. Copyright © 1996-forever by The ISV Foundation. ALL
RIGHTS RESERVED INTERNATIONALLY. Used by permission.
Scripture quotation marked KJV is taken from the King James Version of the
Bible.

Library of Congress Control Number: 2014952805

ISBN-13: 9780989101424
ISBN-10: 0989101428

Printed and bound in the U.S.A.

This book is dedicated to my family.
My children Greta, Sebastian, and Xavier
are my inspiration. My wife Breanne is my
love, and without her little holds together.

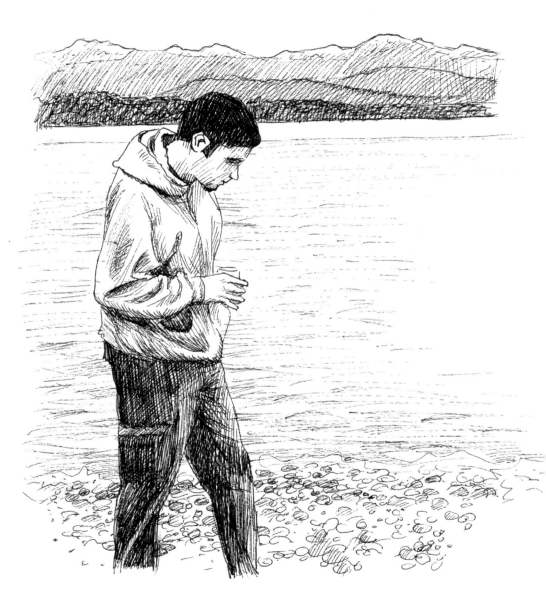

Introduction

The act of seeking is essential to life. When faced with turmoil and struggle, I often take the posture of a seeker. In the following pages I have compiled a series of sketchbook entries that span six years and tell the story of my battles with cancer. I have re-drawn and re-worked them to fit this format; however, the message put forward is intact: This act of seeking was one that revealed a loving God at work when everything in my life appeared to be crumbling.

May 2008

Any time now we're going to be a family of four. I believe we've settled on the name "Sebastian." My little Xavier is excited to be a big brother; he's gonna have a ball. Breanne is ready. We've got things together for the hospital— not that we'll remember them as we rush out the door! I feel ready as well; being a father has been exhausting but so fulfilling. I'm glad I've saved up enough sick days from work in case they're needed.

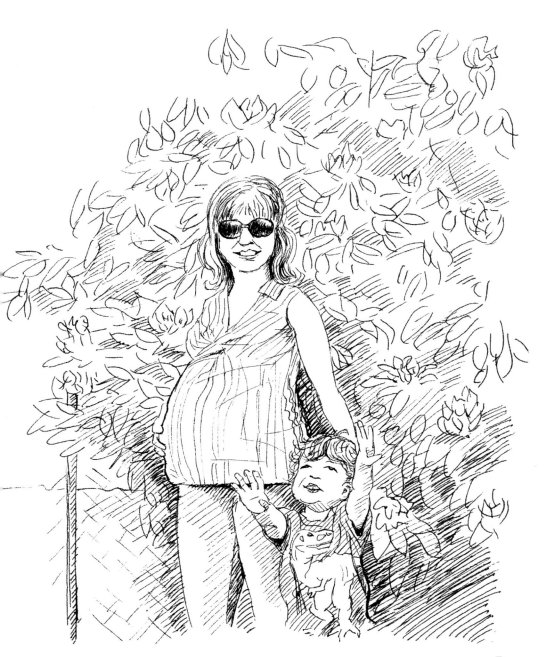

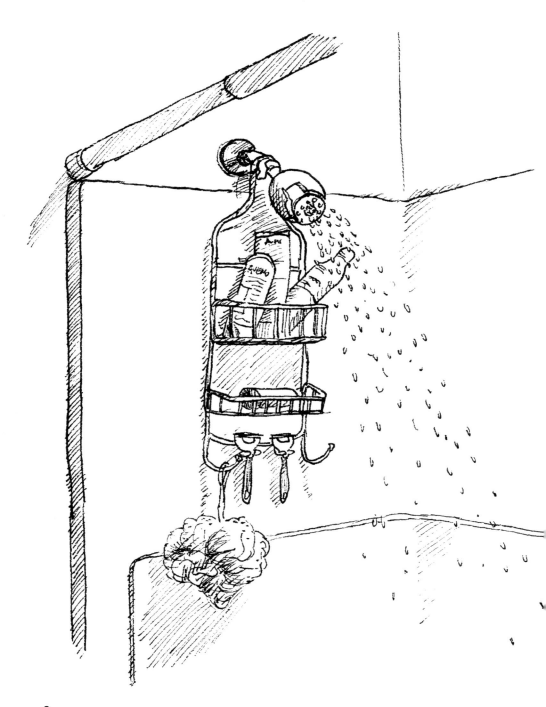

Most men notice when things change on their bodies but they usually ignore it. I've had a concern the past few weeks and finally tell my wife about it. I figure after the baby is born, there will be little time for anything.

When Breanne goes in for her scheduled check-up, I will meet with my doctor to get this concern checked out. I don't really know what to think about it right now.

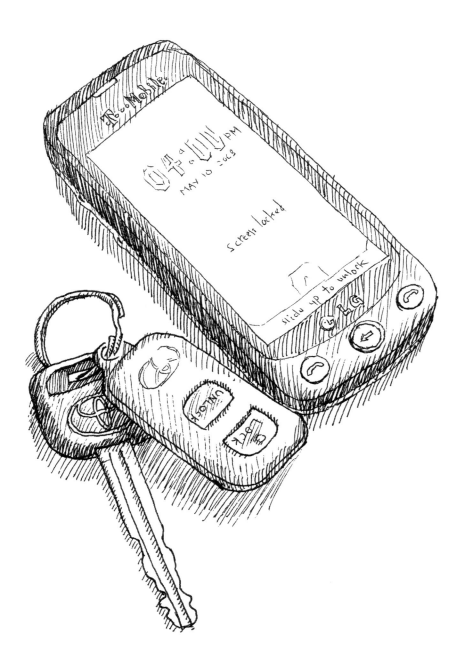

The visit to the doctor's office is strange.

First, my doctor isn't in, so I see a physician's assistant. I get my blood drawn and a battery of little tests, one of which is with the lights off and a flashlight over my scrotum.

Second, nobody is really talking to me. They say things like, "We don't know" or "It's probably not much."

Finally they say, "We'll contact you soon to let you know."

Great. Waiting by the phone sucks!

I wouldn't say that it's anger I feel when I hear the word "cancer." I would describe it as a deep disappointment, that I am letting my family down at a time when they really need me. I don't like the attention that it brings me. And breaking the news to friends and family is difficult on many levels.

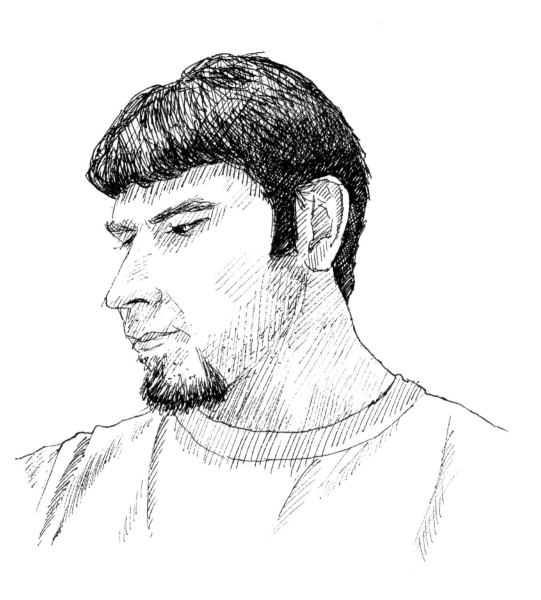

From the low of finding out I have cancer to the high of becoming a father for a second time, I am feeling rather dizzy!

Our new member of the Fraley family arrived safely and in good health. He also arrived quickly: less than an hour and a half at the hospital and he was born. My wife's plan of having an epidural and taking it one step at a time was quickly turned down. Her dilation was already at 10 cm when first checked.

Sebastian was born one week after my orchiechtomy; so all of us are in recovery mode following this amazing day.

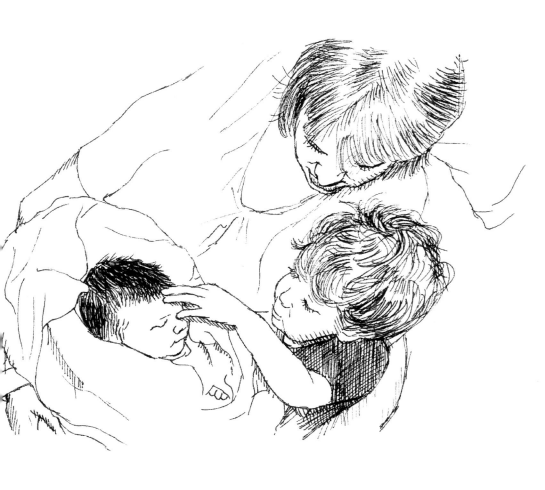

Thank you, Jesus, for staying beside us
during these eventful days!

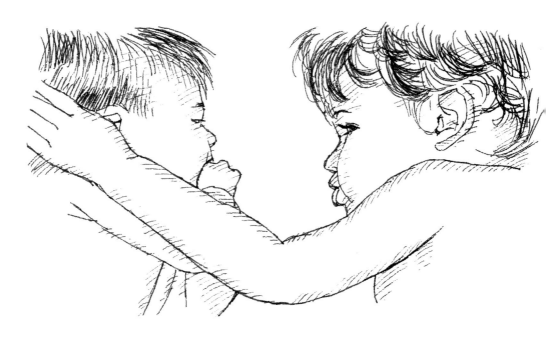

June 2008

Two brothers. One of those moments full of joy. They're lying on the floor side-by-side, just a couple weeks since I found out I have cancer.

And at this moment I know I can heal. I don't exactly know how; I just know it is possible.

Watching them inspires me to face any challenge. The word cancer loses part of its sting, even though I know it won't be easy to travel this path.

After meeting with the urologist, we are offered 3 treatment options:

1. Watchful waiting

2. Retroperitoneal
   lymph node dissection

3. Chemotherapy

My wife and I
do some research,
spending time
online, asking
family and friends,
and praying. This is
one hard decision!

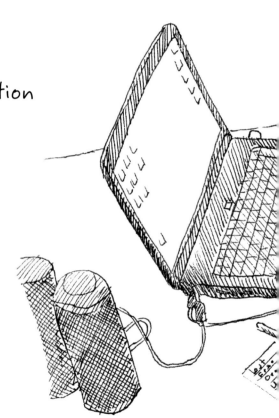

We settle on #2, the RPLND. This is the one the doctors most recommend. Now to plan when it will happen.

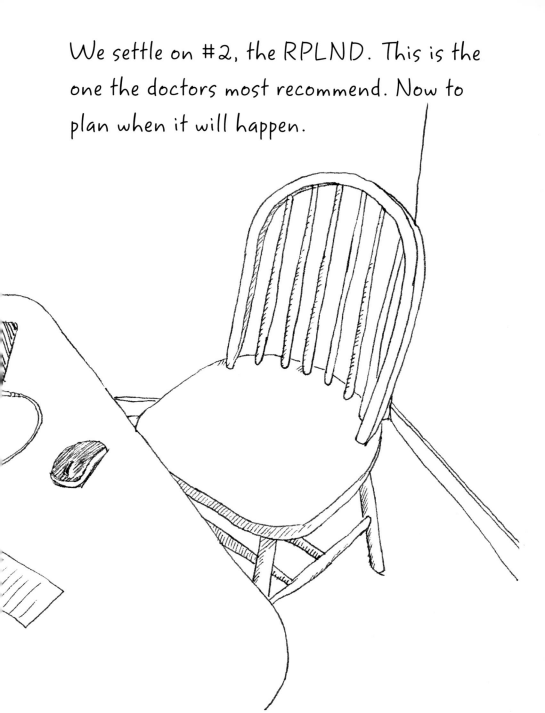

August 2008

Ready for the road!

After setting a date for the big surgery, we
make the decision to visit family in Idaho
and Colorado. I'm excited to have an
adventure that will hopefully keep
my mind from being stuck
on cancer.

It's a
3,000-mile
round trip

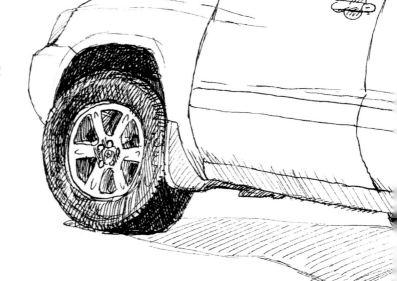

from our home in Seattle, rather adventurous
with an almost 3-year-old and a newborn.

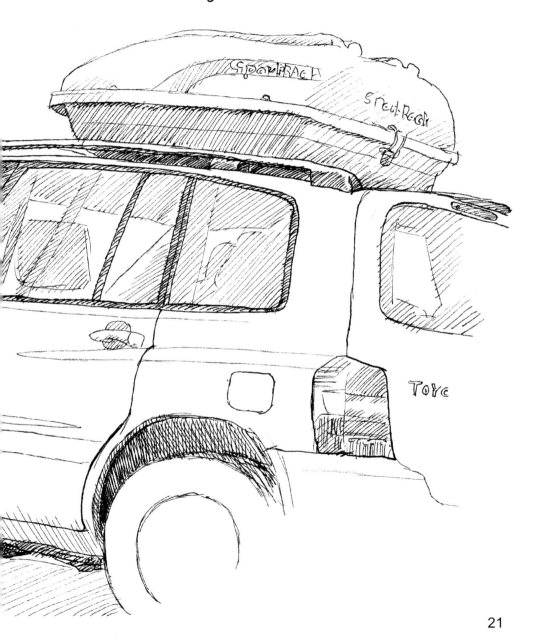

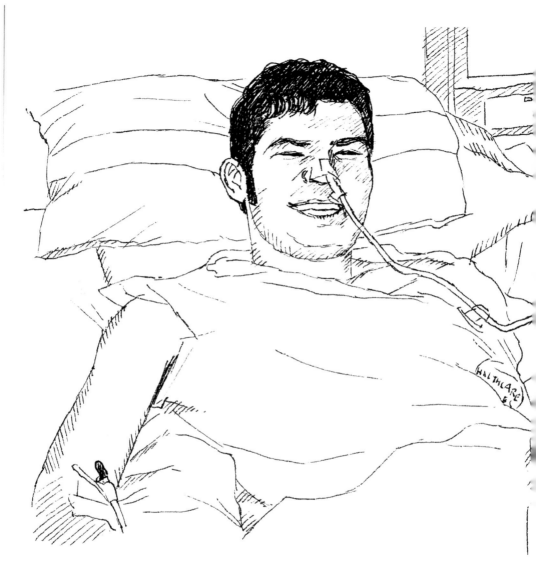

August 2008

Hard to describe what it's like waking up
following surgery. My RPLND was a

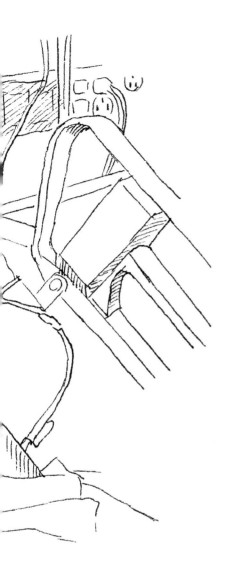

success, no cancer found in the lymph nodes that were removed. As the pain medication wears off, I begin to feel the extent to which my body has been invaded. I can't really pull myself up; it feels like I have been filled with cement. The incision that runs from below my belly button to my sternum is bandaged heavily; I almost mistake it for a pillow. The NG tube makes itself known by the discomfort in my throat. Despite these unwelcome guests, I smile. The road ahead looks clear.

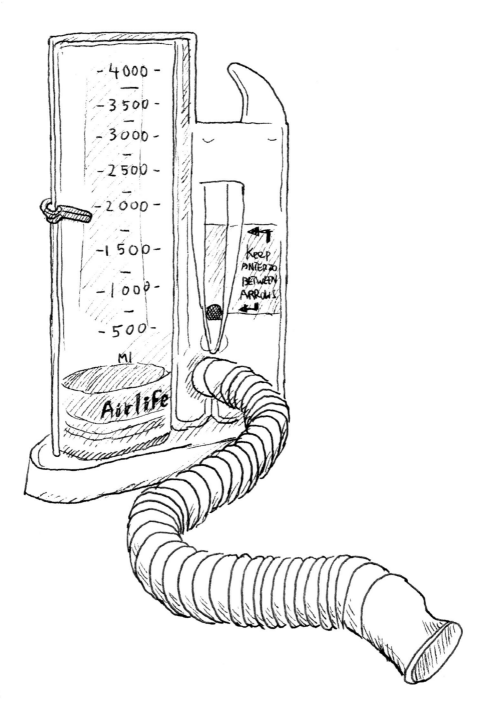

The Volumetric Incentive Spirometer
is not a pleasant device. It sits on my
side table beside my hospital bed
and all I have to do is look at it
for my giant bandaged abdomen to
recoil in pain. I am supposed to exhale
and keep a floating measure between
the designated arrows, and do this
repeatedly throughout the day. Yes,
my lungs enjoy better functioning.
But right now I just want to push
fast-forward on my life.

The hardest part about being stuck to a hospital bed is not being able to pick up my son Xavier when he is close to tears. He doesn't want to be here, his eyes are avoiding mine, and his body language says, "This isn't right. It's hard not to have my daddy."

After my family leaves, I cry — not for myself — but for this forced separation and the pain it is causing them.

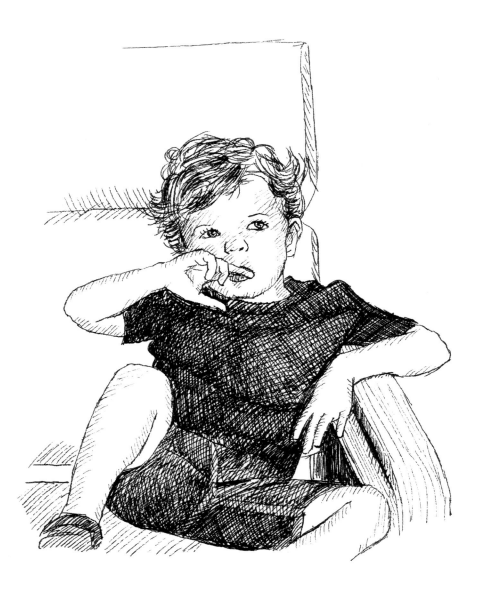

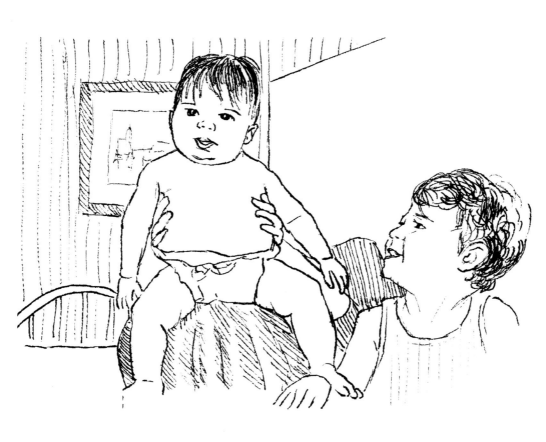

October 2008

Life is slowly returning to normal. It's Halloween, and the boys are having fun with the pumpkins that are ready to be carved. I actually haven't thought about cancer the past few weeks, only when other people bring it up.

My back is finally feeling straight. It no longer feels like I'm having to strain to keep my chin from falling into my chest. Work is going smoothly. Teaching my class has been fun and challenging (special education is different every day, and I love that!).

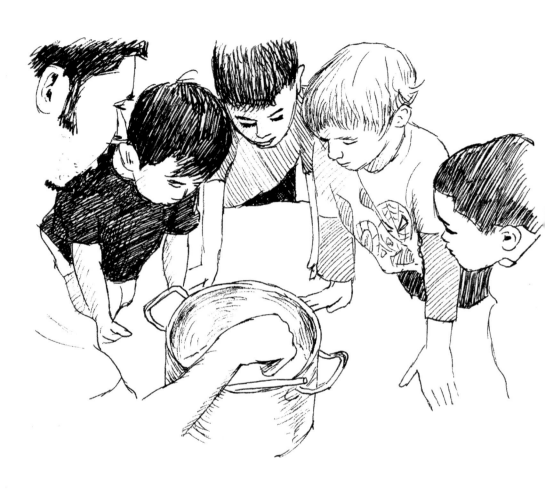

February 2009

Teaching preschool special education is a blast. I get to play guitar, cook, build things and destroy things, run outside, create cool stuff out of recycled materials, etc. ... I could go on for a while.

The tough side is dealing with strong behaviors, all the tedious paperwork, long meetings, that hopeless feeling of herding cats (what it feels like some days!), and seeing the effects that abuse and dysfunctional families have on children.

Overall, it is an amazing job, and I am thankful for it.

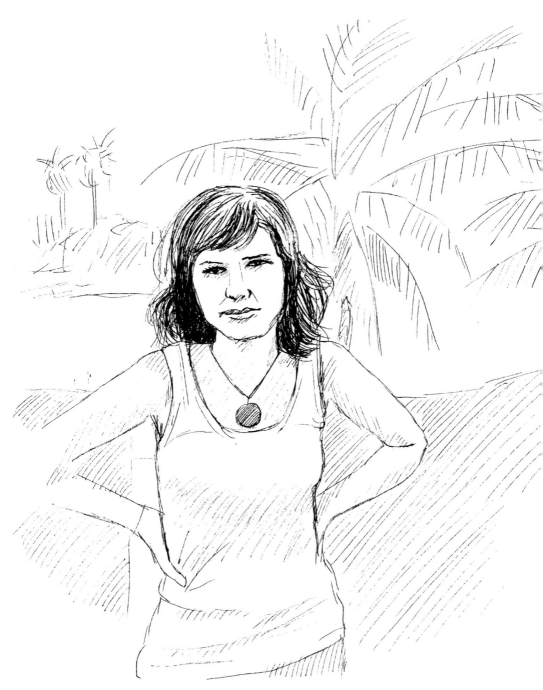

June 2009

Fortunately, I don't get this look from my wife very often. She's beautiful in all that she does and a little part of me giggles when she gets so upset. Doesn't help the matter, but that beauty and anger just do something to me!

We're enjoying a vacation in Mexico, and despite what I've sketched, we're having a great time, a break from our crazy routine and busy family life.

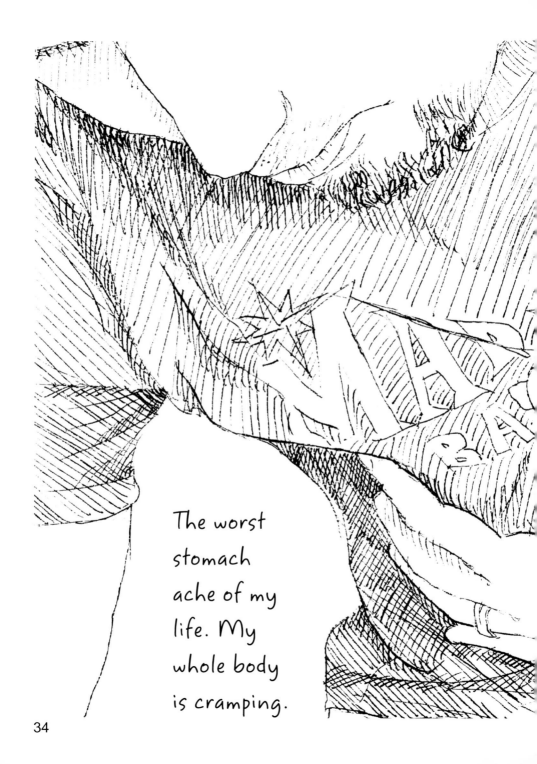

The worst
stomach
ache of my
life. My
whole body
is cramping.

I've taken Tylenol, Ibuprofen, whatever else and absolutely no change! In fact it's getting worse. ...

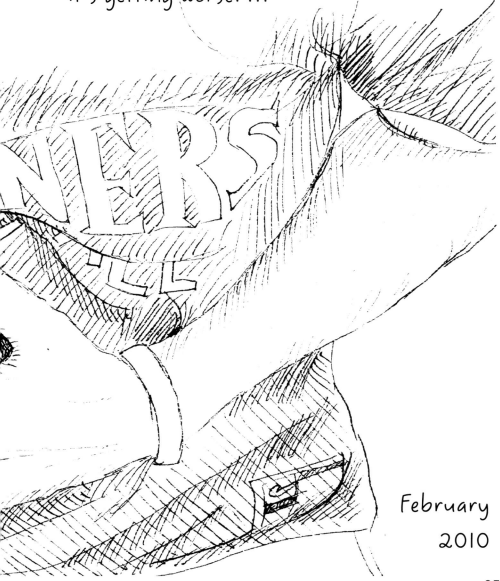

February 2010

After unsuccessfully waiting out my stomach ache, I finally decide to go in to Urgent Care late at night. My friend Hans drives me there.

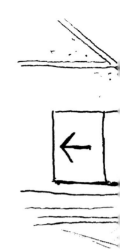

The cramping is unending. I get more meds, stronger ones. I am told a number of things, some of which anger me: "You might just have the flu" or "Are you sure it's not a reaction to gluten?"

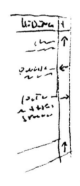

Despite the pain I go home several hours later to see if I can sleep any. Fat chance! The next day, still no change.

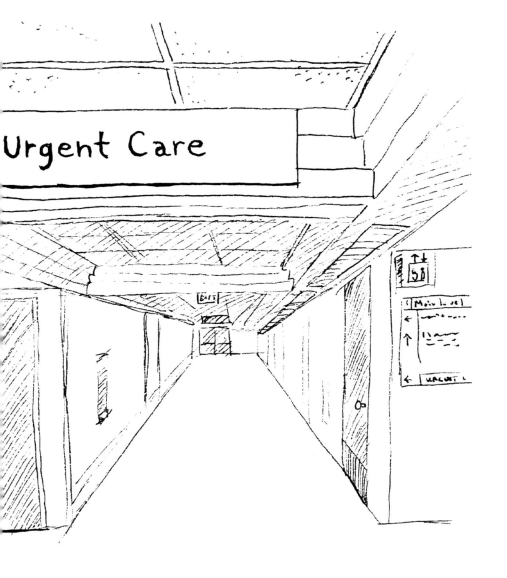

I go back to the clinic close to home,
and the doctor there suggests it's a
bowel obstruction.

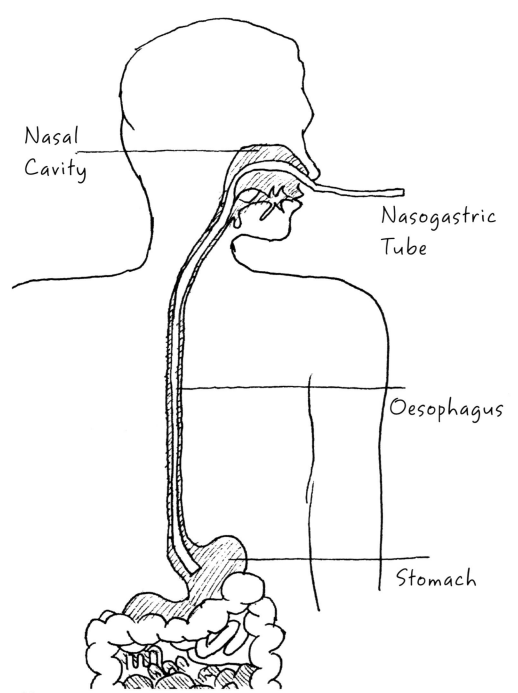

Nasal
Cavity

Nasogastric
Tube

Oesophagus

Stomach

Apparently, the scar tissue from my RPLND took over my abdomen and decided to block passage in two places. The doctors say it's like rubber bands that keep looping over until it completely constricts. That explains the stomach aches!

The first measure taken is to send a Nasogastric tube to my stomach to provide a way for the excess bile to be suctioned out.

I hate it!

I hate it with a passion.

More doctors come in. I feel something is up. They aren't talking to me yet, just murmuring and looking over charts. Great! In my mind I'm picturing more rubber bands.

I am not ready to hear what they are sharing. In fact, I feel like I am watching the scene from outside my body.

Two lymph nodes are swollen on the back of my abdomen, and blood tests reveal the cancer has returned. It is growing again.

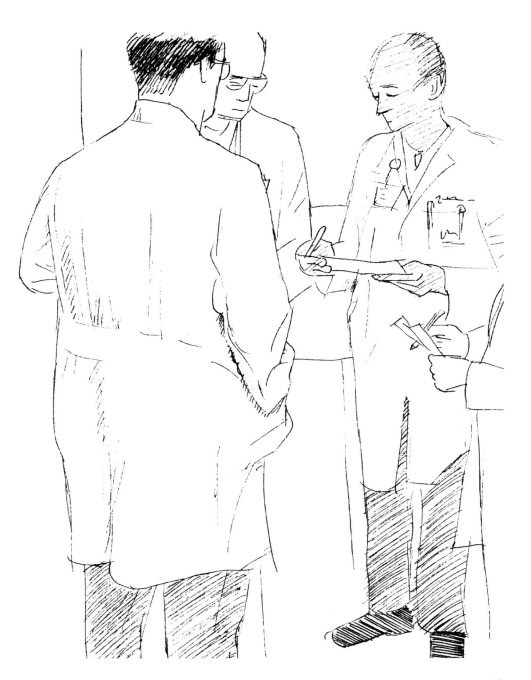

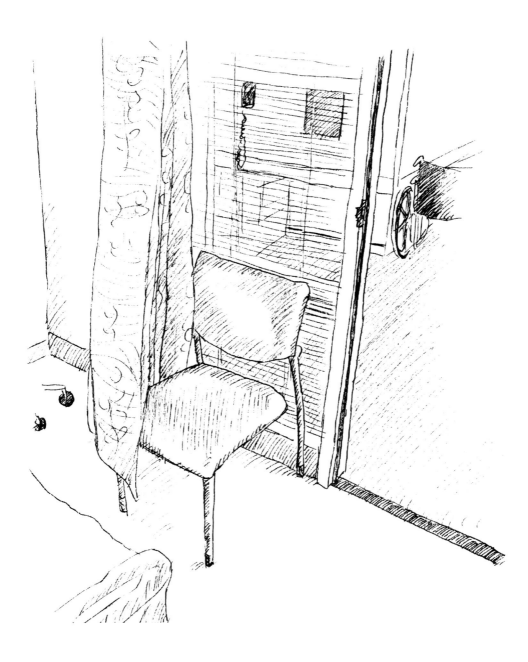

After surgery to clear the bowel obstruction, I wake up in the post-op room with intense pain. The person beside me is asking questions and all I want is to be numb. I need more pain medicine.

Soon enough I'm wheeled up to my room; and I realize that, for the next 6-10 days, this is where I will be. The next morning I am helped up out of bed to stand for the first time. I'm dizzy, nauseous, and in pain.

That empty chair feeds my loneliness.

There's no button on this stupid remote that can get me out of here. Again, I am overwhelmed by life that is deciding to throw me under the bus. I cry and find no reason to stop.

This breakdown is mental and physical; there isn't much lower than this feeling.

Dear God, I know you love me and care for my family. But what am I supposed to do with this? Is there any other way to do things without pain involved?

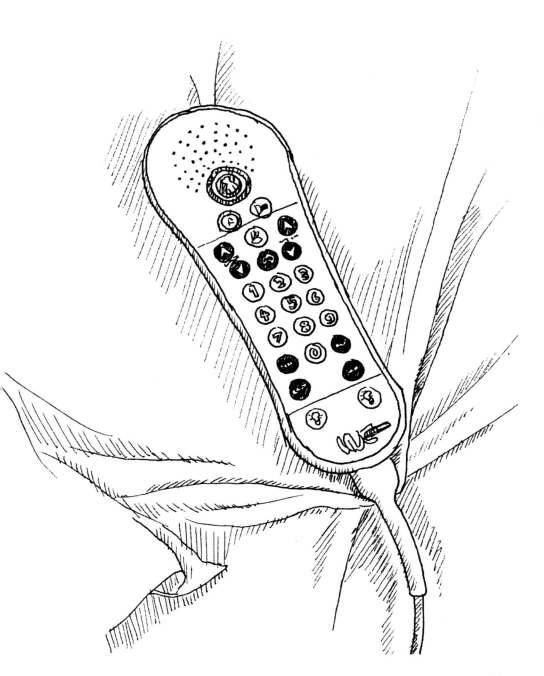

Jim Manker is the first person to make me laugh following surgery.

He looks over at my NG tube, as it is moving bile and other things out of my stomach, and asks the people in the room if anyone wants a peanut butter and banana smoothie. I'm thankful for something to laugh about.

But more than that, Jim's heart and passion, his eternal enthusiasm, and his readiness to bring a word of hope, make me feel loved.

He's the type of person you need around when things are hard, and a dark cloud hangs overhead.

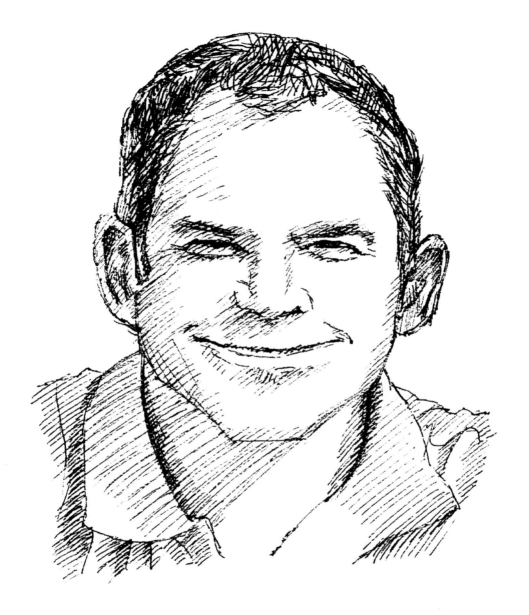

Jim is my pastor at church, and he keeps my
faith alive by simply showing up and making
me laugh.

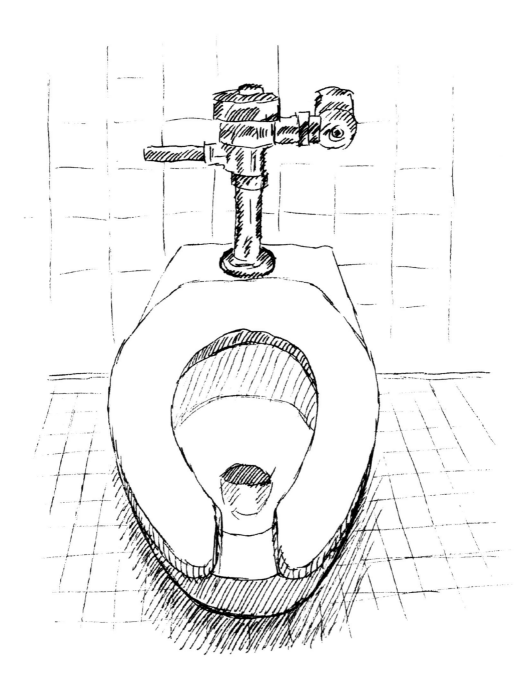

Going to the bathroom after major surgery of the abdomen is an experience I would never wish on my worst enemy.

The fact that once I am able to fully go, I may be released to go home, just adds to the pressure and anxiety.

I can't ever recall having prayed for poop before, but now I am pleading, practically on my knees. All I can manage is a whisper of gas. Guess that's a start!

March 2010

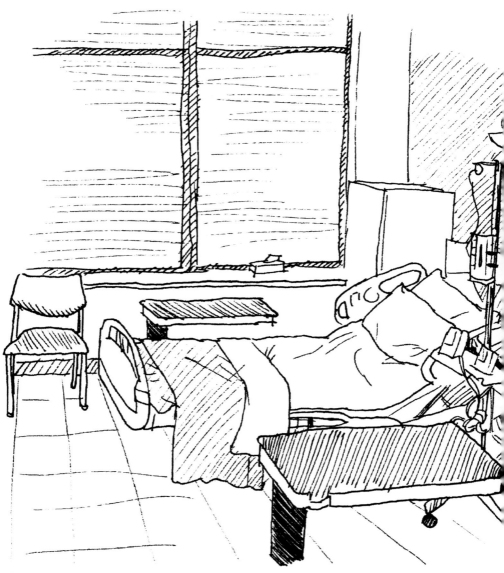

After a short 3 weeks of recovery from surgery,
I begin chemotherapy at my home away from
home, the infusion center
on the 5th floor of the
hospital in Seattle.

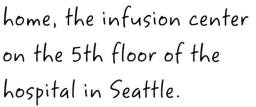

I am given the extensive
rundown of what it means
on a day-to-day basis,
and I am introduced to the
drugs:
Cis Platinum
Etoposide
Bleomycin.

My schedule is set: one week on
and 2 weeks mostly off. 3 cycles.
Basically, 9 weeks I'm dreading.

I return home from my first day of chemo.

My mother gasps when she sees me. She swears I look like a ghost. All the fear and apprehension of this experience is scaring the crap out of my blood cells, apparently.

My mother has seen me sick many times growing up, but never this way. I reassure her I will be OK.

Just wish I could convince myself!

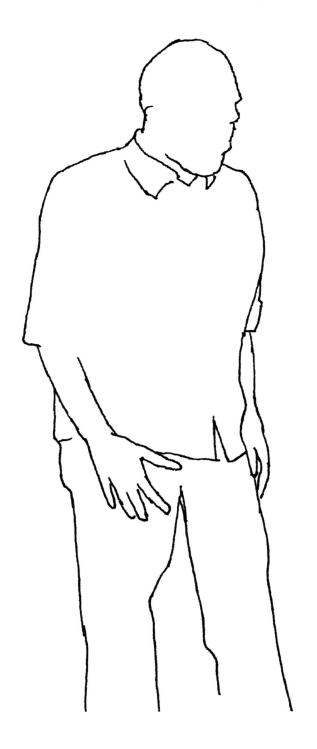

At Green Lake enjoying a
beautiful spring day. I'm
wrapping up my first week of
treatment. I'm doing OK
trying to get a hold on things.
Each day is different, hard
to know how I will be feeling
from moment to moment.
When my energy is up,
I want to go and use it,
take a walk or see friends.
When it's not, I want
to crawl into a shell
and disappear, wait
for this slow
anguish
to pass.

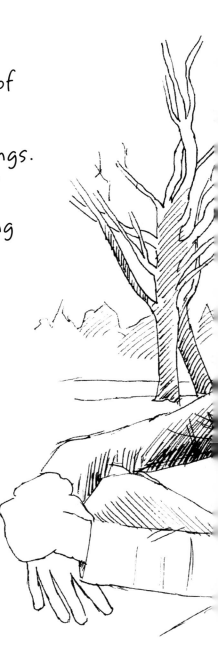

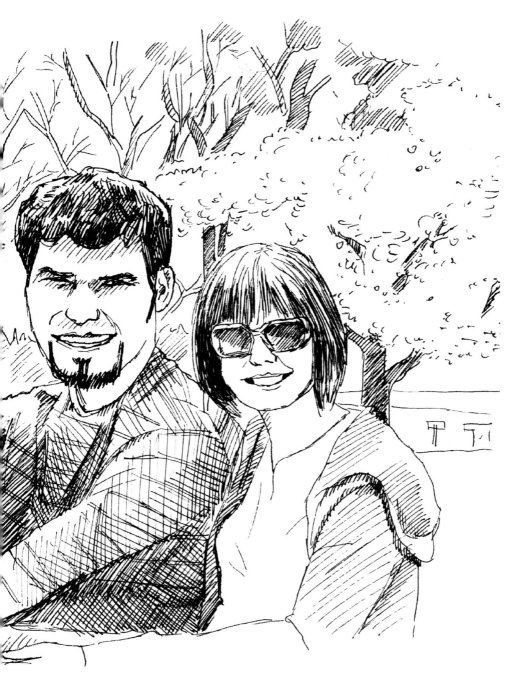

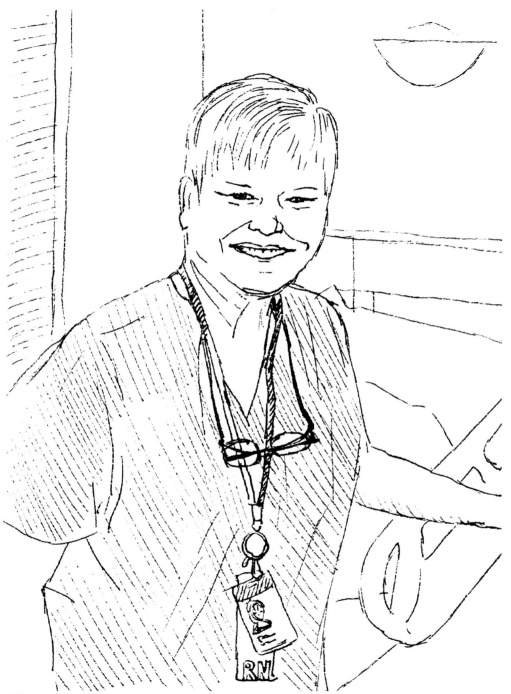

Karen is my lead nurse. From day one at the infusion center I have felt comfortable with her.

You can sense the breadth of knowledge she carries, but her most impressive quality that stands out is her kind and reassuring delivery. She just makes you feel safe, like nothing is outside of her control.

I am fortunate to have her beside me when few things feel normal.

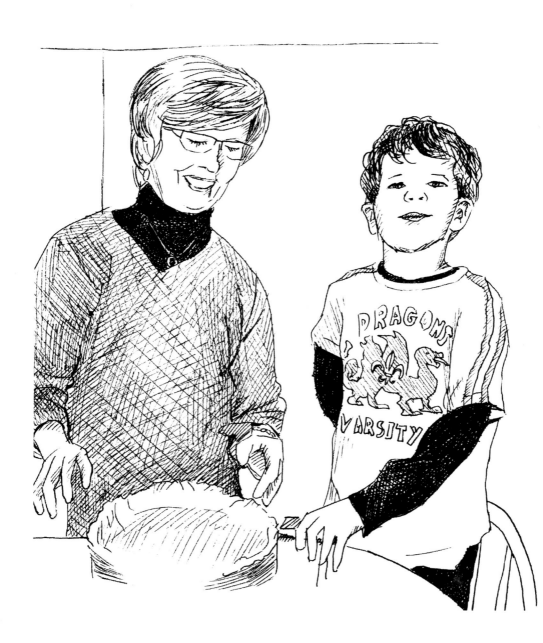

April 2010

For a cancer patient, an act of love
is to take care of their family during
hospital stays or treatments.

My mother, Carolita, pulls out the
recipe book and gets my Xavier to bake
a pie.

This time spent together, when I am
unable to do much, brings me comfort
and reassurance. I worry more about
my kids than about myself, even though
I am the one who is sick.

April 2010

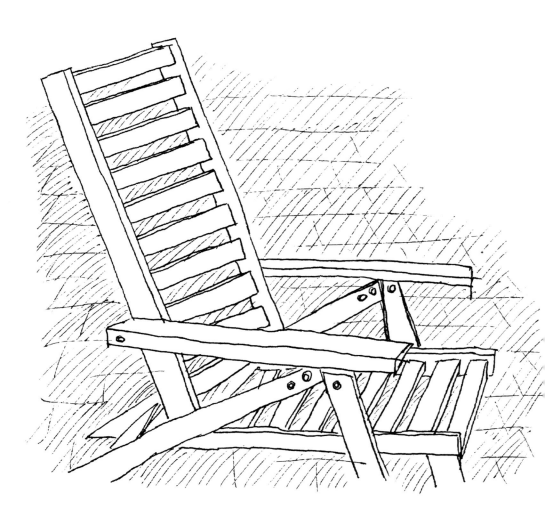

I am drawing my neighbor's lawn chair on a decent April morning. I feel OK and want to take advantage of that feeling! I don't know when it will be back again!

Our neighbors, Chris and Greg, have been so kind, even though they may think it's a little strange I'm drawing their lawn chair in my PJs.

Each line connecting the slats to the frame is giving me a satisfaction that is difficult to describe, other than that I feel alive and capable of something, even if it appears insignificant.

There's a sadness that exists, and you recognize it when you're honest.

Cancer makes you honest and helps you see you can lose what you hold close.

That sadness is not all bad, for it guides me to Jesus and he speaks:

"I love you and I know it hurts. Put your faith in me."

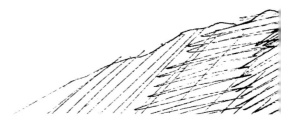

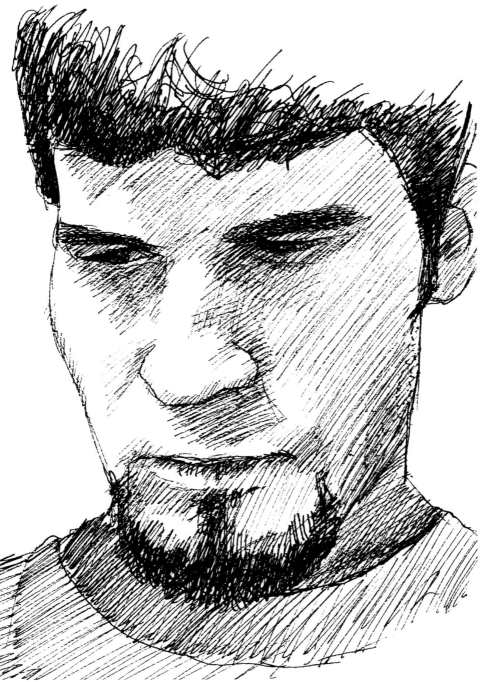

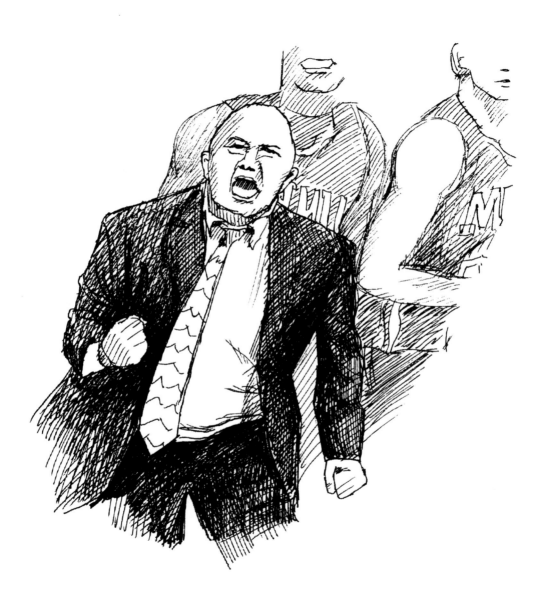

Dear Coach Lamar,

As I sit here in a hospital bed getting my chemo treatment, I look back on the time when I was a basketball player at MNU. You were a tough coach, and I sometimes disliked the hard work you put me through! But with more understanding and greater perspective, I have come to see how your influence in my life has been tremendous. First, I learned to become tougher and more resistant, like a fighter. Second, I learned to quit making excuses for mistakes, and move forward. Finally, I learned to see how a relationship with Christ is what true life is about. Your life has impacted mine immensely. Love you, Coach. You're helping me fight this ugly disease by what you taught me.

~ Mark

Breanne and I were already in debt when cancer hit. I panicked several times, just thinking about what might happen. My brother John stepped in and became our bank. His reassurance helped me to focus on my health and not worry so much about the endless parade of bills. His incredible generosity brought peace to our family in this area.

Check if address is different then the billing

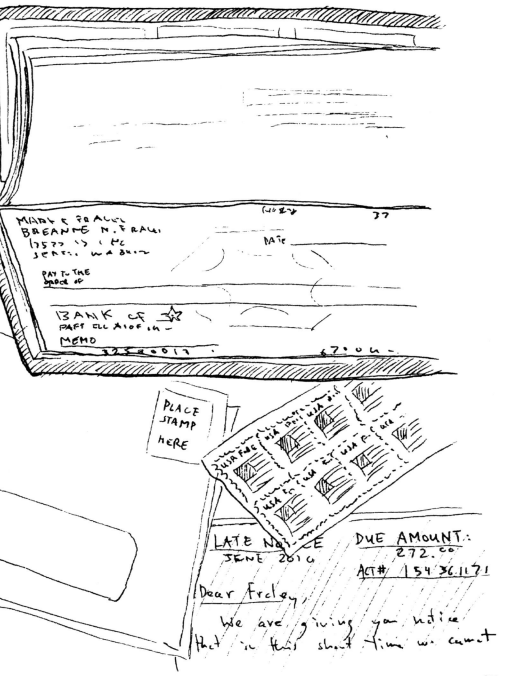

May 2010

During chemo, my activities
include:
   put on sweats, lie down
   on couch, watch TV, play
   some computer games, lie
   on couch, nap, occasionally
   walk outside, go to bed.

It is hard to focus on
anything for more than
5 minutes. I don't enjoy
reading or, for that matter,
drawing. I only keep drawing
because I know it is a part of
me I refuse to lose.

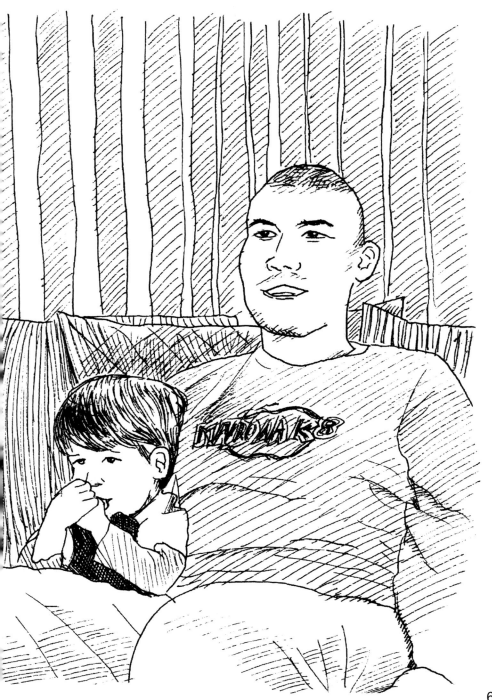

My mother-in-law, Susan, has stepped right in and brought her fun and enthusiasm to my boys in a much-needed way at this time.

Her caring spirit and the way she gets them to be silly and playful, tickles my heart. She is such a genuine person who gives of herself all the time.

I just pray that this rubs off on the boys, and in turn they can love those around them, in need or not.

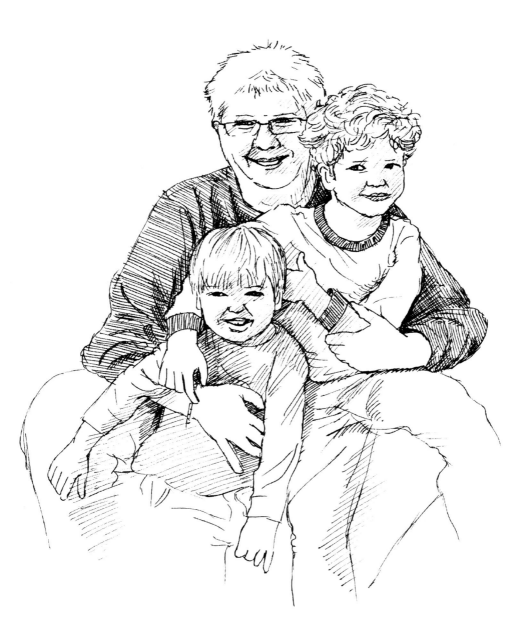

71

Jerre White is a long-time family friend, and just the other day I received from her an inspiring gift: a 48-piece set of Faber-Castell Pitt artist pen brushes.

I immediately got them out and sketched away.

This gift is timely. My frustrations with the inability to focus or concentrate have been ruining artistic output. These pens are bringing creativity back into my life.

Thank you, Jerre. You may not know, but your gift is remarkable.

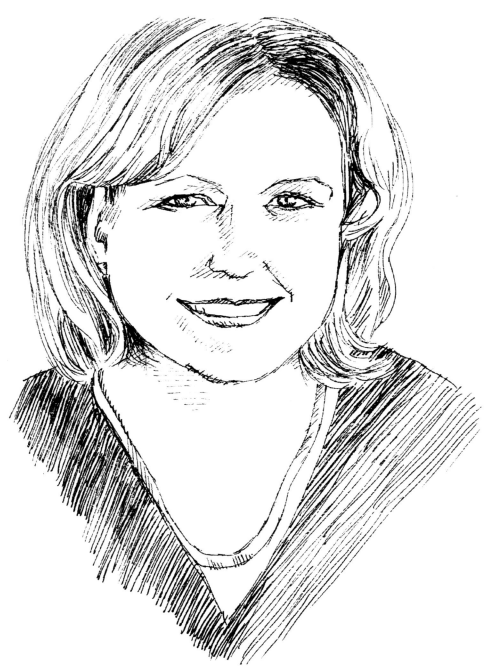

73

I have gotten to know my medicines rather well.

The pain killers are necessary, but when taken too much, I'm constipated and my night sleep suffers. The anti-nauseas are rather harmless, and I have had success with those. My favorite happens to be Lorazepam, an anti-anxiety/nausea drug that has helped me sleep better and made me feel better overall.

It's funny writing about my favorite medicines; before all this craziness, I rarely even took Tylenol.

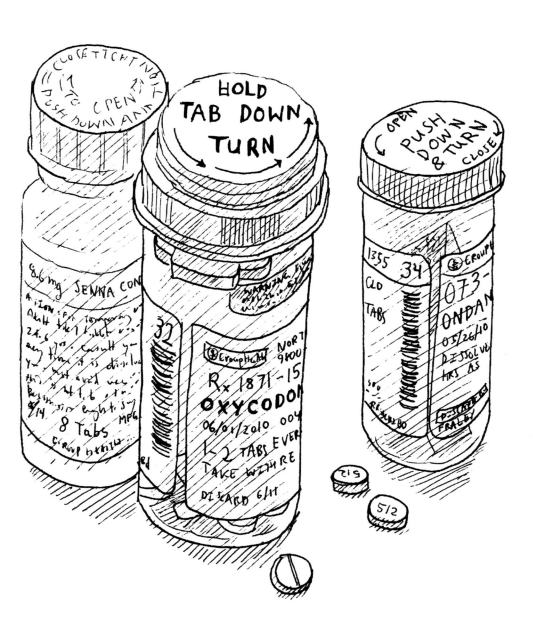

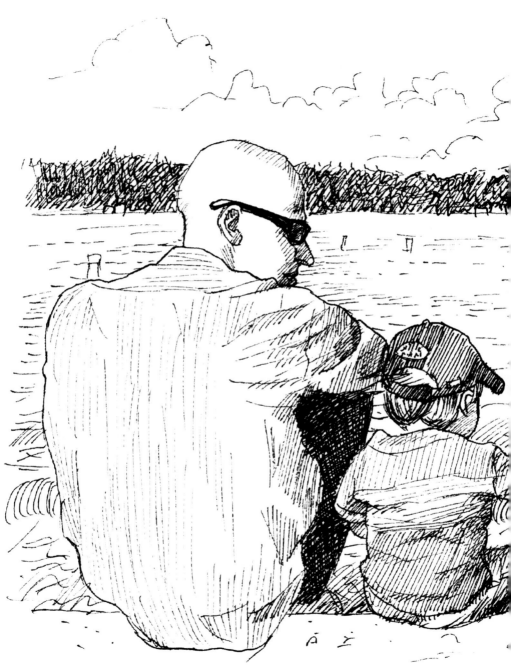

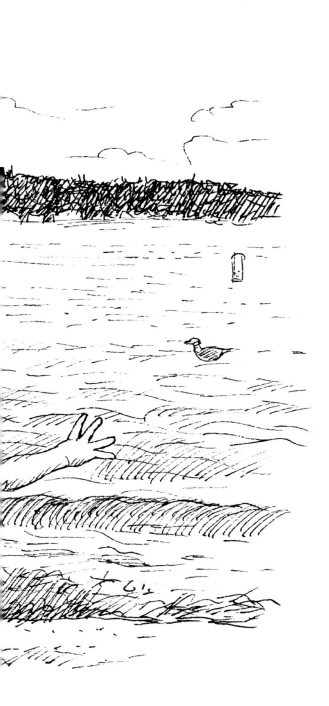

Following my last treatment of chemo, Sebastian and I sit and watch the ducks at Matthew's Beach. We enjoy the moment of calm and peace. This moment turns into hope, a hope that is reachable and lasting.

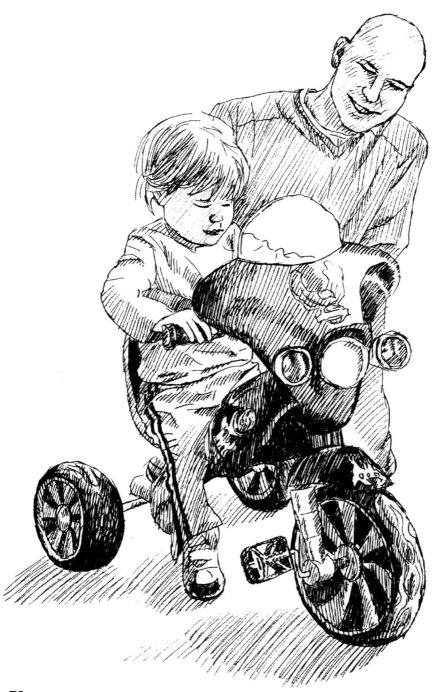

I believe children hold a certain healing power. Not in a magical way, but rather in a calming, peaceful way.

My son Sebastian receives a cool tricycle for his birthday. As I watch his reaction of joy, happiness, elation, and amazement, some of it rubs off on me.

My children provide me with a strength that is needed to move forward. I can forget my condition when they are with me.

I often hear people say, "Children are a gift from God." And now I have a better understanding of those words.

I'm so lucky to have this woman by my side! Her inner strength rivals any small nation's army, and she brings me to the realization that the important things in life are right in front of me:

faith
family
friendship
(and good food, as she's
 a great cook!).

Cancer has made me more aware of what an incredible woman she is.

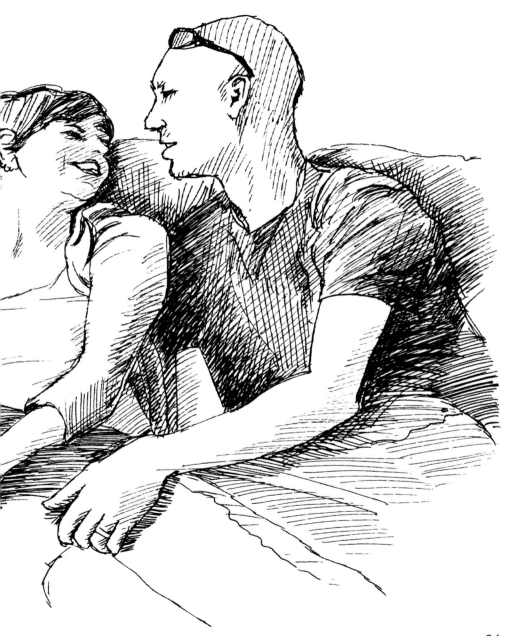

June 2010

The weirdness of cancer: cool to have
a shaved head, not cool to have absent
eyebrows.

I honestly don't think about my look
too much. I've accepted it. When my
family looks at me, they see ME. ...
That's all I can really ask for.

Drawing this portrait feels strange, as
all my standout features — excessive
eyebrows, sideburns, goatee, and moppy
hair — are only there when I close my
eyes.

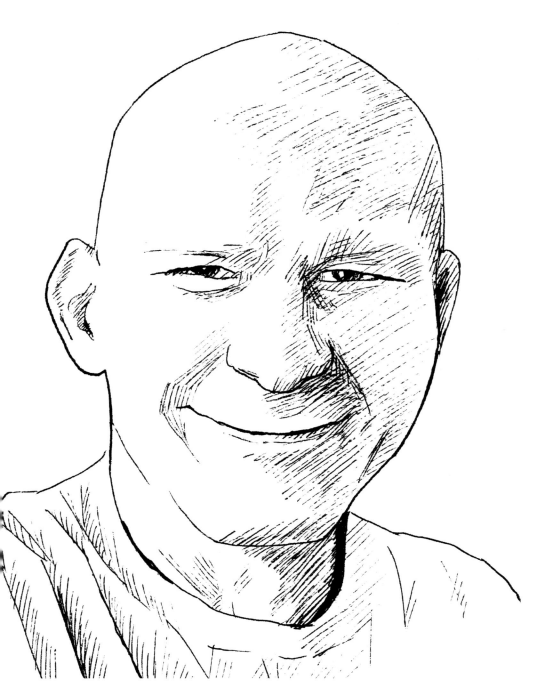

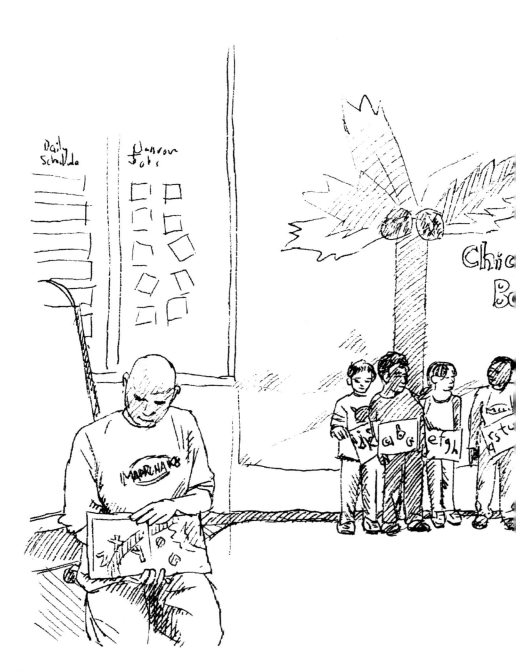

Back to work. Sure feels good.

My students are getting over the bald head thing pretty quickly.

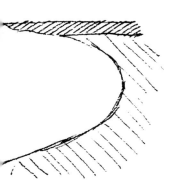

Teaching is something rewarding, something I feel good at from years of experience. It's just what I need to feel productive and useful again. My energy isn't all there, but my co-workers are the best, and they step in when needed.

Returning to work also avoids our having to pay COBRA insurance, since I came back just within the 12-month Family Leave Act limit.

My long-time colleague, Fertis, in the preschool special education classroom, is my role model for strength and courage. She takes the toughest of the tough and softens their hearts, brings them into community.

I take the example of how she lives her life and apply it to my struggle with cancer, never backing down, but leading from the heart.

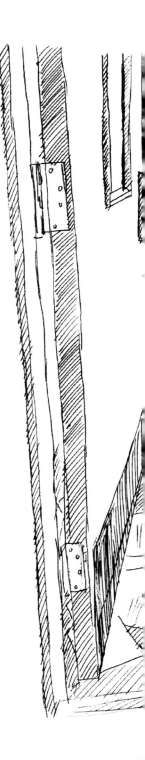

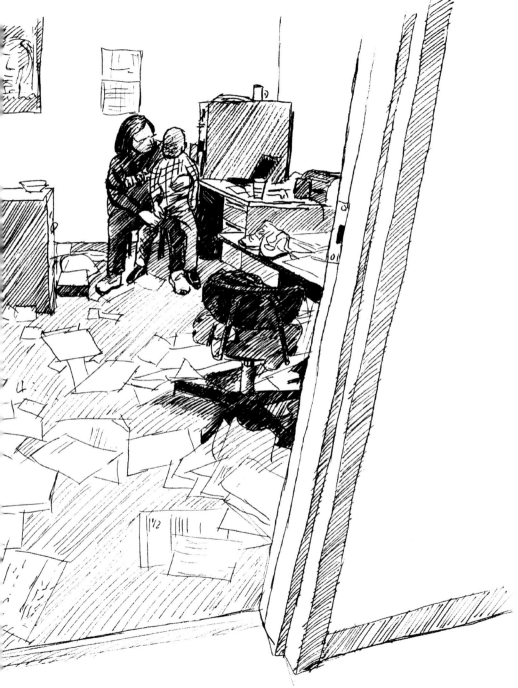

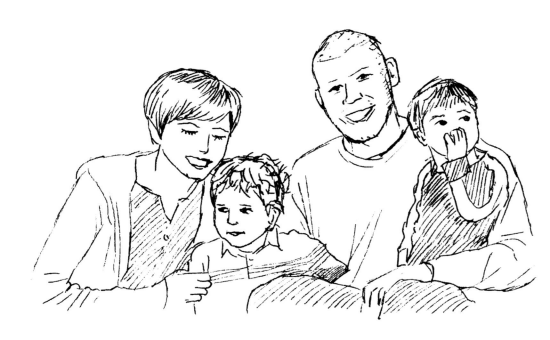

Trying to do things as normally as possible is important, even if it means taking horrible family pictures. We are usually pretty photogenic, but I have to say each time we try, the results are rough.

My hair is just now growing back, and I am most excited about having eyebrows again. I missed them, even though I lean more towards a unibrow. I haven't shaved in I don't know how long, so the little bit of stubble above my upper lip and on the tip of my chin has me rather excited, feeling manly again!

We're gonna keep snapping those pictures until we get it right.

July 2010

Hans and I jam away on a summer afternoon, out in front of the house. This moment is good for the soul, because it's tied to freedom of expression without any constraints;

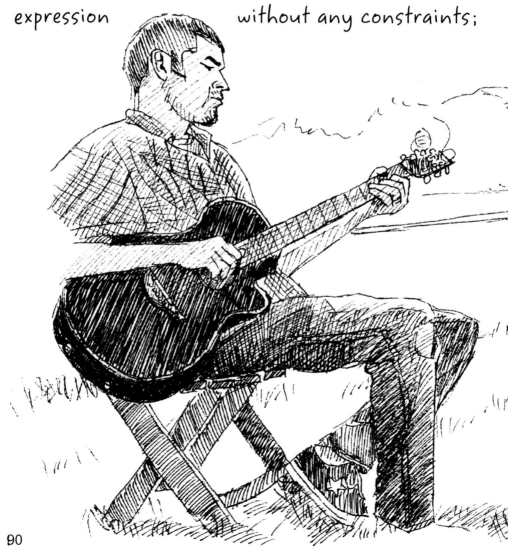

there's room to be creative and to breathe.
God protected my body, for
which I am so thankful; he
also protected my spirit and
soul.

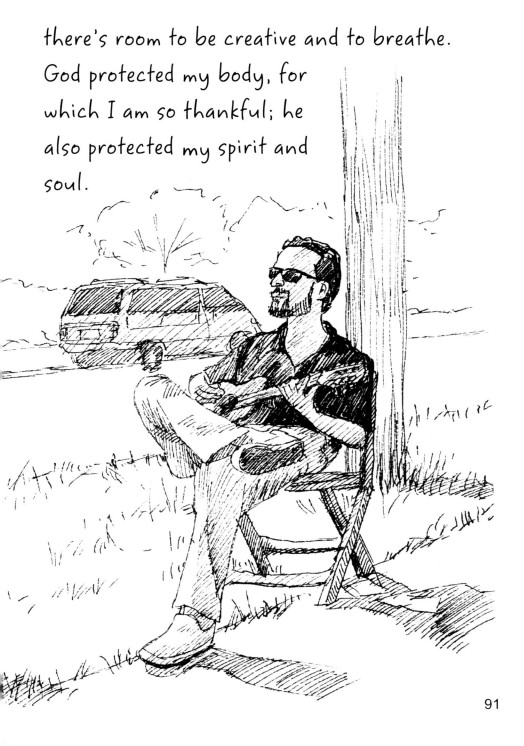

August 2010

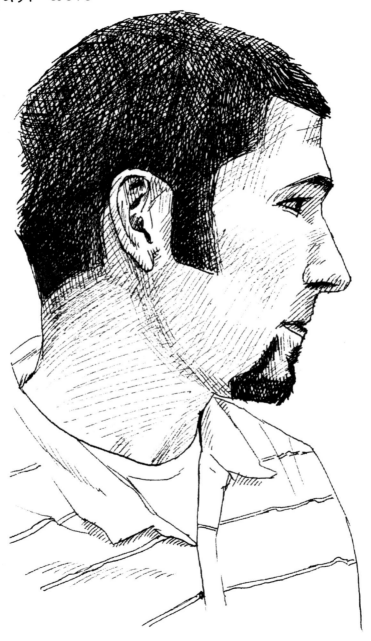

My love, Breanne. What would I do without you? I love our relationship, the playfulness and deep friendship, the honesty and commitment. You are the one who keeps this family together during all the craziness. You are an astonishing woman!

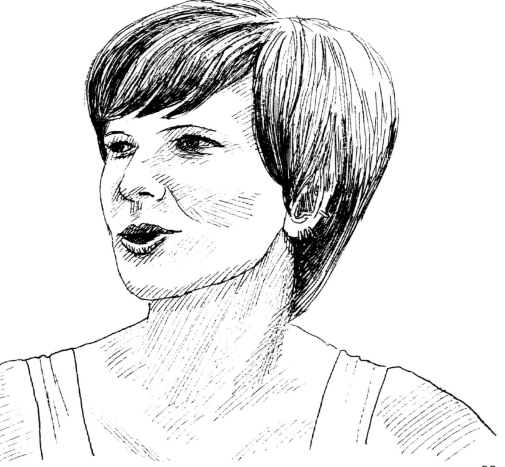

We take a hike at Wallace Falls, about 5 miles long with a lot of ups and downs. Sebastian rides on my back and shoulders most of the way. Good test of strength and resolve.

My body feels like mine again, not belonging to some cycle of drugs or to some medical need. I can make it hurt of my own choice, a good kind of hurt, one that makes me feel fully alive!

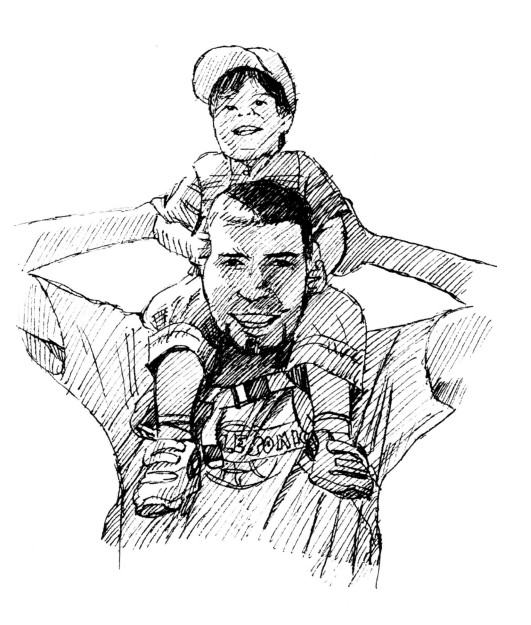

October 2010

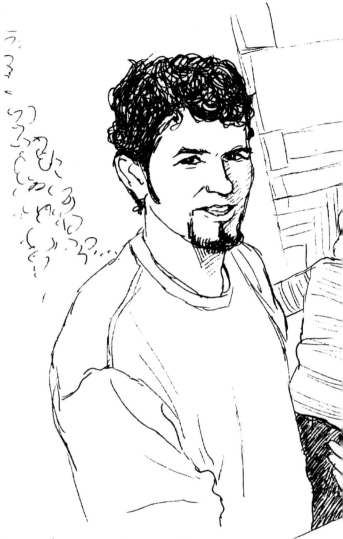

Family life, not much more to say!
My hair is coming back in differently.
For the first time in my life, it's curly —
and extremely soft.

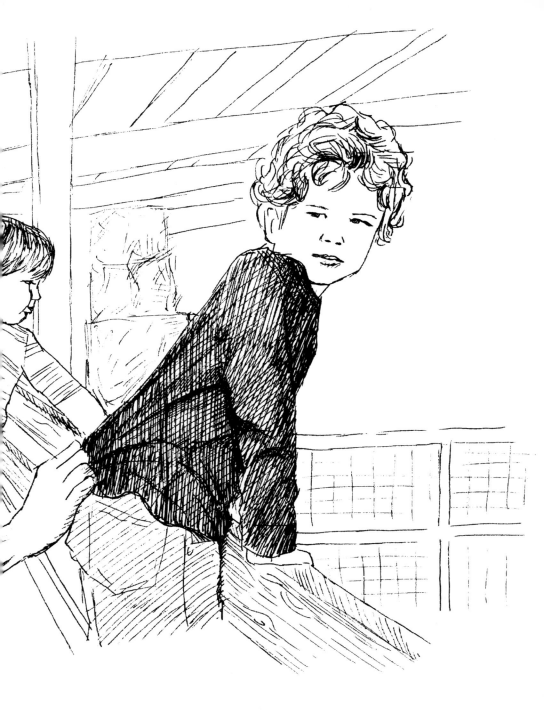

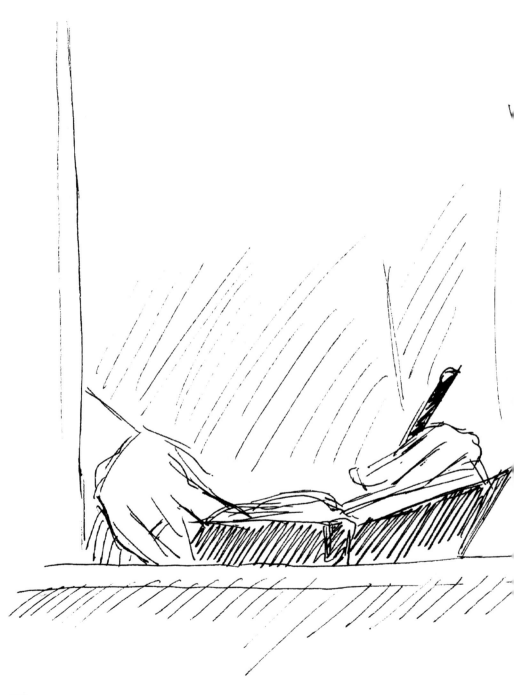

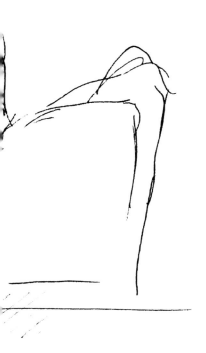

Sketching my reflection
on the opposite window
in a near-empty bus. It's
early in the morning,
I'm on my way to work,
and I'm engaged in the
creative process. My
mind is focused, my
thoughts connect, and
ideas begin to pour out
as pen touches the paper.
I feel a steady, calm
energy that courses
through me.

June 2011

Out of nowhere another stomach ache gets the better of me. There really is no warning to this one, as I have felt fine for a long period of time. Sure enough, that same cramping — that I feel even in my back — has me going straight to Urgent Care. Before any scans or tests, I know what it is: another bowel obstruction. I'm prepping myself for several days of misery, when on the hour or even half hour I am throwing up. The worst is the tube that runs through my nose and down to my stomach and gives me absolutely no chance for rest as it clears my stomach of any accumulating bile. It is my life nemesis, an enemy to my spirit, even though it is physically a helping agent. I can't even draw it, as I want nothing to do with it.

I have hit rock bottom.
I'm heading to Virginia
Mason by ambulance,
my bowel obstruction
hasn't relented despite
3 days of hospitalization.
I've thrown up countless
times and feel at the end
of my rope. Physical,
mental, and nearing
spiritual
exhaustion.

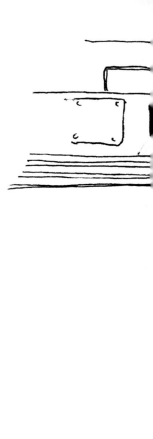

I feel empty
in a broken way,
where my person
has leaked through
onto the ground.

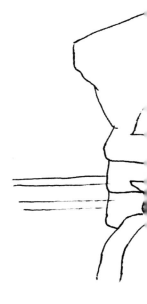

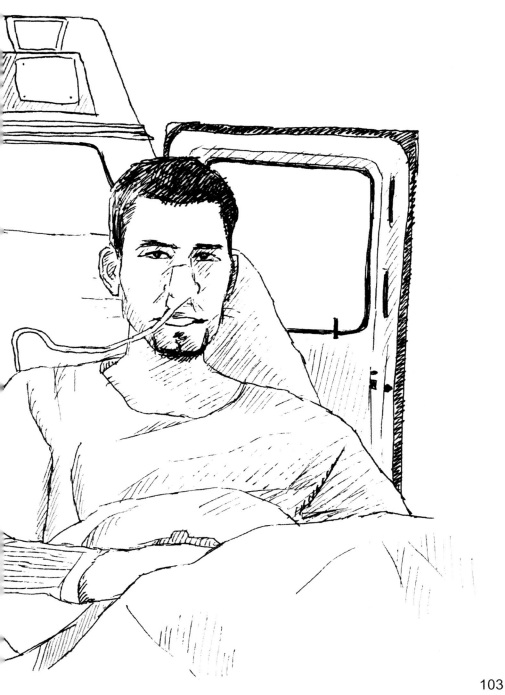

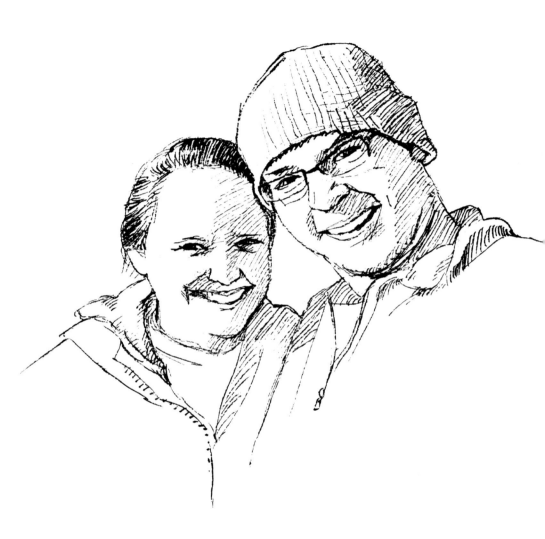

My good buddy Jason Harwood and his wife, Stephanie, have been true friends. I am broken and feel my lowest ever. Just before I head into surgery, Jason prays over me for God's protection and for His care over my family. Tears flow out as I release deep-rooted anguish and sorrow. My body shakes, but I feel safe to let it all go.

I believe that's what a true friend can do: be there in the moment and speak truth or allow truth to happen.

The boys do their best to smile following my surgery. Xavier is looking to the side, avoiding eye contact. It hurts him to see me like this. Sebastian is reaching for a smile, but it looks strained; he's trying too hard.

I feel ashamed, in a way, that I put them in this situation.

Dear God, comfort them! I can't right now.

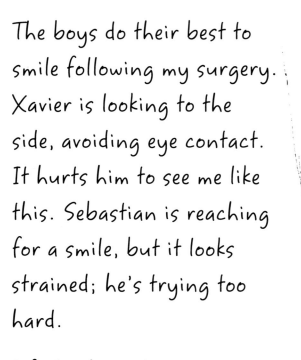

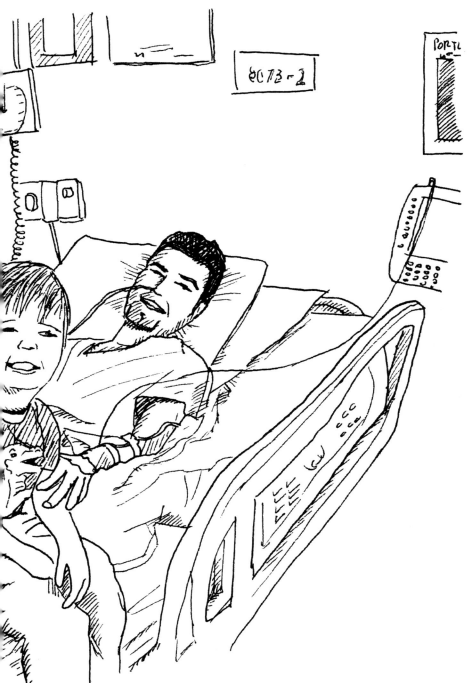

Breanne has carried our family on her back, doing everything to keep the family happy and together.

I'm pretty much worthless right now, but I am able to see just how much Breanne's love filters down to every aspect of our life, from sunset to sundown.

She loves and continues to love.

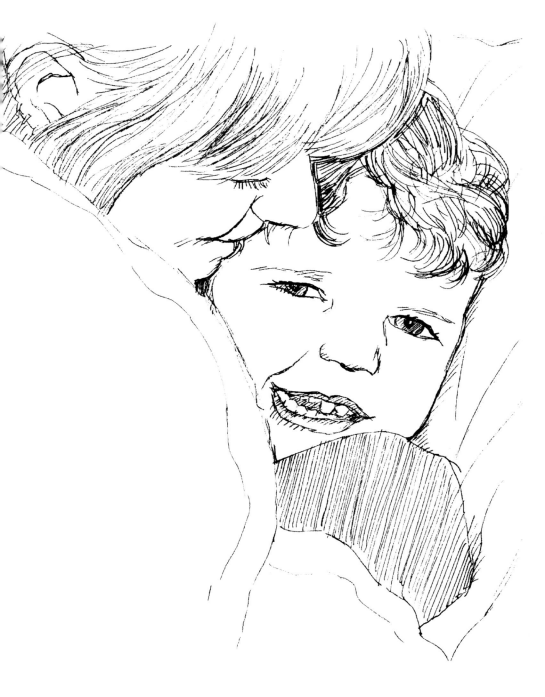

I would like to think my cancer has pushed my art forward and brought to it a confidence and honesty that was lacking previously. I was a copyist before cancer. Now I AM AN ARTIST. I have something to say, to share with the world. I have things to say so that they do not stay trapped inside.

Dear God,
please guide my steps into this strange arena of creating art that reveals things about me.

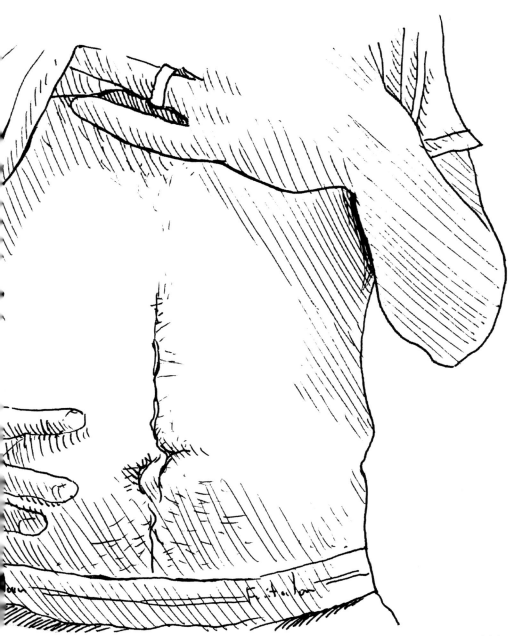

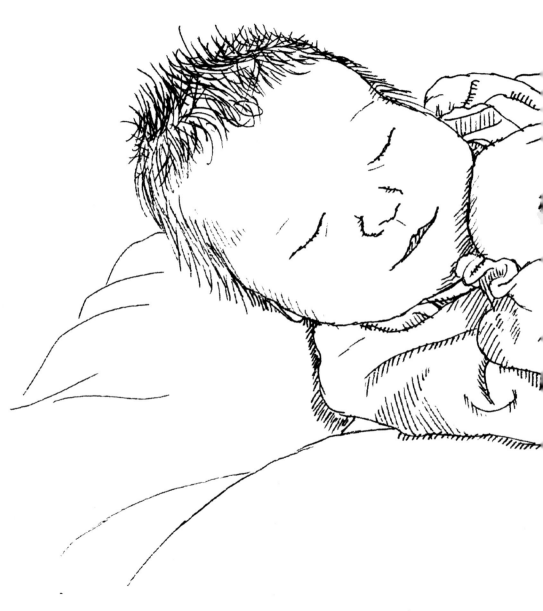

November 2011

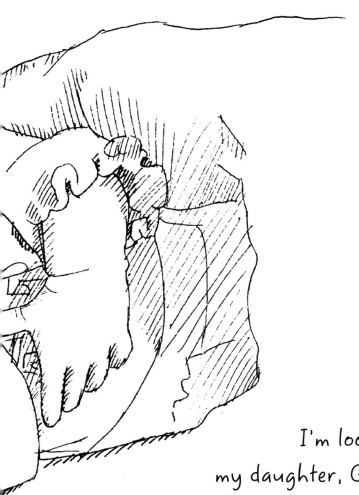

I'm looking at
my daughter, Greta Jane,
and wondering in amazement
how she ended up in my arms following all the
surgeries and chemo I have been through. She's a
a gift from God, as cliché as that may sound, and
I am so happy for the joyous torment she brings
into my life. I am one lucky daddy!

December 2011

Breanne and I stand in the hospital elevator and joke about having a punch card for hospital visits: "Your 10th trip is free, on the house!"

You have to keep a sense of humor to stay alive and, considering our recent adventures, it's amazing we've made it this far. My body has tried to kill me 4 times (testicular cancer, bowel obstruction, cancer, another bowel obstruction). That's a serious case of bad luck or just God's weird way of saying, "You can handle a lot!"

I'm ready to exit the elevator.

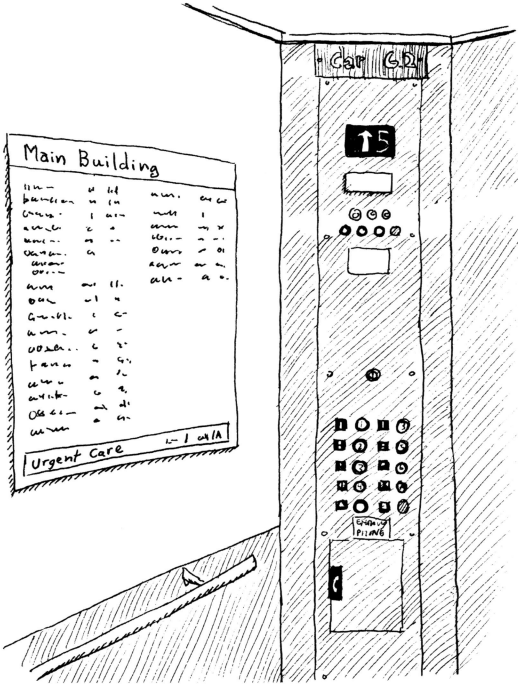

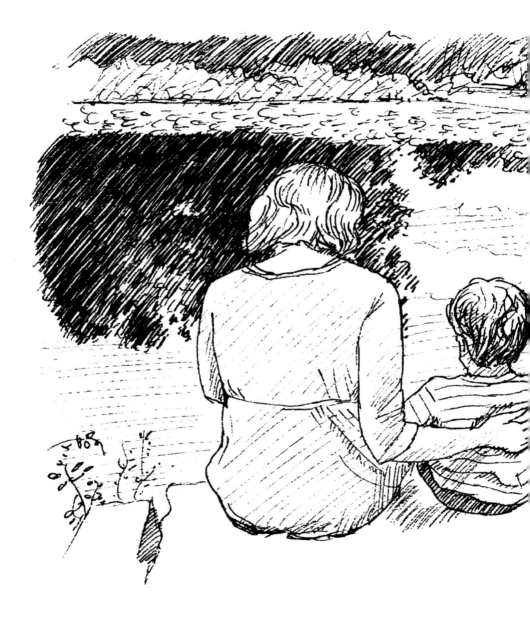

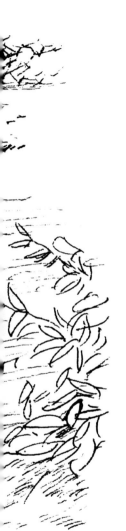

I don't want to say cancer taught me anything. Cancer is crap; I will never give it any credit.

Instead, I can say that I was broken by cancer in order to be rebuilt in a different way through God's help.

I have a different posture, have learned to reflect, and now can see the beauty in small events or moments. I have always been "artistic" but never dug deep enough to explore the emotions and feelings behind it all. That door is now open.

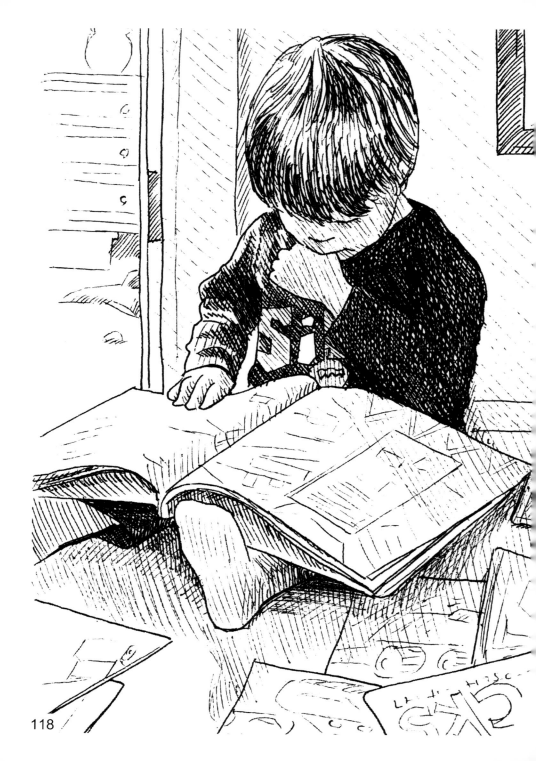

As an adult, I look for images that make me pause and want to look closer.

This particular image starts a creative fire in my mind, leading me to represent more the emotion I feel than the lines and values found in it.

I connect with the feeling of being a father, of my son immersed in books, in the quiet calm of a lazy afternoon, in a moment of childhood that can only happen in childhood.

We are on Camano Beach,
turning over rocks to watch
the tiny crabs scurry about.

My son Xavier is a nature
boy and a natural explorer.
He could stay out here all day
without a second thought.

I hope that this fascination
with the physical world will
transfer to the inner world,
and that he discovers a God
at work in him, who loves him.

Keep looking under those
rocks, Xavier!

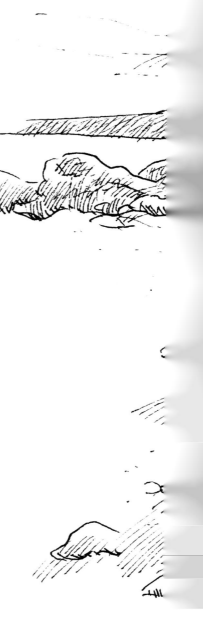

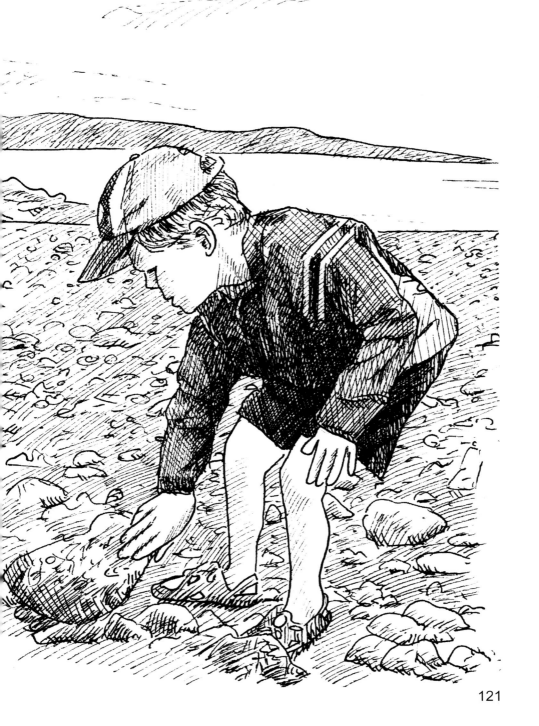

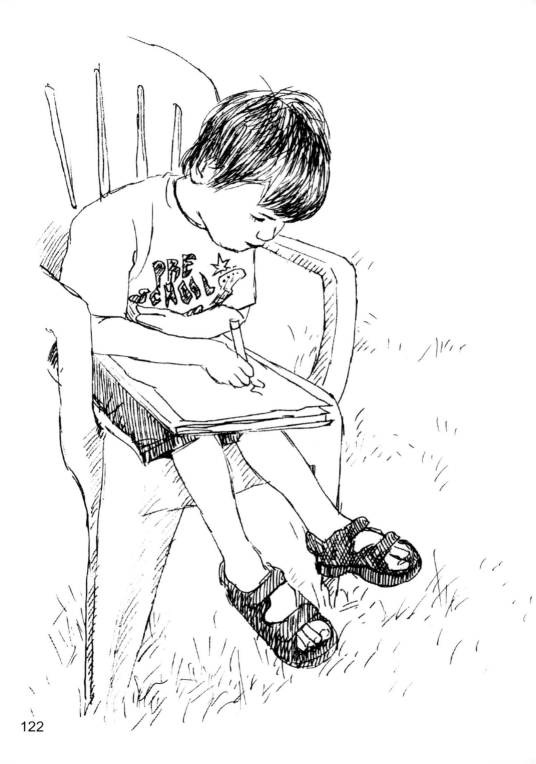

One of my great joys is to watch how my children each engage in creative output.

My middle child, Sebastian, is a true artist. He takes his drawing seriously and pours himself into it. Long stories flow from the marks on his pages. This time ninjas meet snakes who drive fast cars in the pouring rain!

I wish my mind could be so free at times, in full immersion.

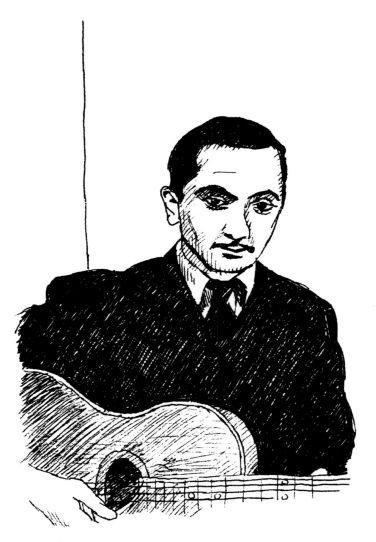

DJANGO
REINHARDT ——————————

This sketch may seem out of place in a book about cancer, but this early 20th-Century guitarist has been an inspiration to me for a number of years. His music, his passion for life, his living in the moment with absolute neglect for tomorrow, and his striving despite all odds, speaks to me on a level few can.

As a young man he was badly burned in a caravan fire in which he lost the use of two fingers on his left hand. He innovated a new technique and played all over the world.

March 2013

I draw with abandon now, taking my
sketchbooks with me wherever I go.
To me, it is a form of meditation.
I often get lost in the moment, and
on occasion miss my bus stop, when
immersed in quiet thought.

Jimmie Valvano has a quote: "If you
laugh, you think, and you cry, that's
a full day. A heck of a day. You do
that 7 days a week, you're going
to have something special."

The "think" part is my drawing,
now an invaluable part of my life.

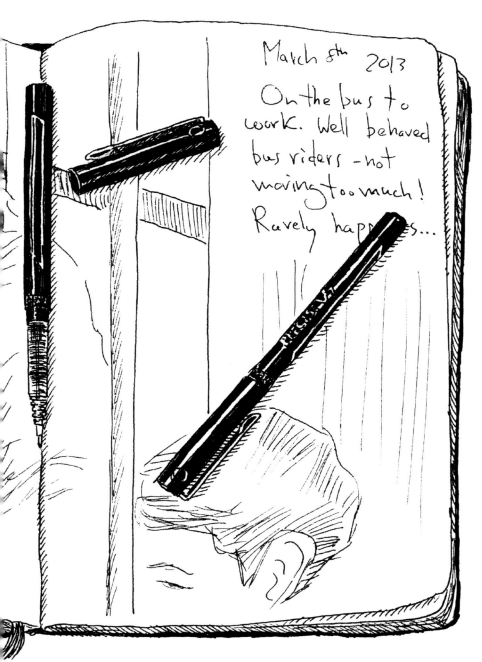

March 8th 2013

On the bus to
work. Well behaved
bus riders - not
moving too much!
Rarely happens...

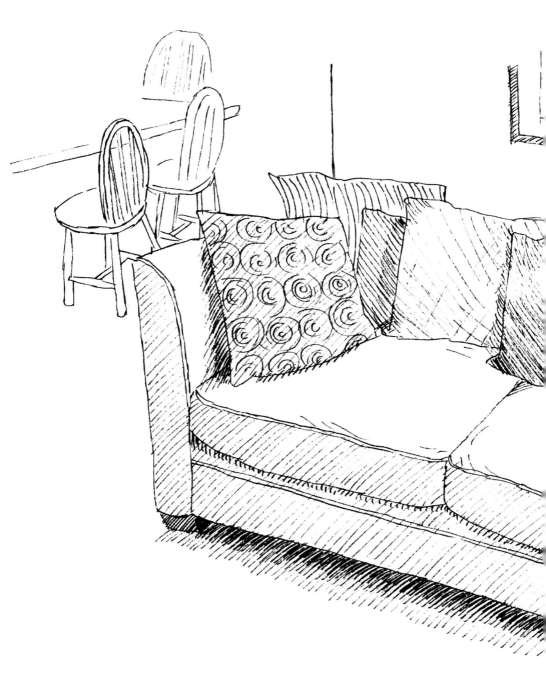

March 2013

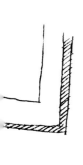

I look at my living room couch and think of all the times I spent with her, curled up and wondering when I would feel good enough to jump up and shake this whole cancer thing. She's a reminder of both the burden of sickness and the quiet transformation that occurs when peace and calm take over, as they move slowly but surely to bring a new day, a new life.

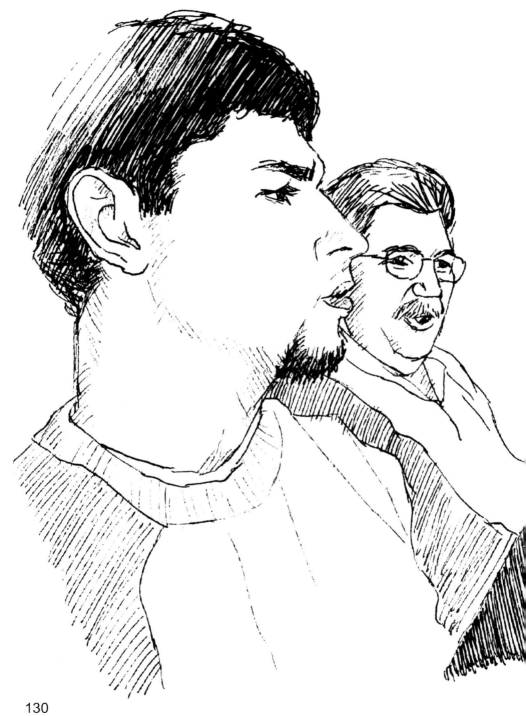

I'm reflecting on this conversation with my pops at a Royals game a few years back, both the moment and the image, and how my pops has shaped me. The more I think about it, the more I miss this dialogue. I need a lot of help in my life, and my father's wisdom has always spoken through the noise.

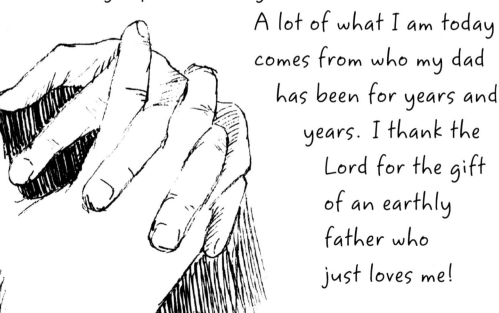

A lot of what I am today comes from who my dad has been for years and years. I thank the Lord for the gift of an earthly father who just loves me!

My brother John is someone I look up to with admiration. He is one of the rare people with a deep intellectual understanding but a kind and thoughtful heart. His analytical ability does not hide his warm side. He's my big bro and I'm proud to be his brother.

My brother Matthew is a man of his word; he is honest and loyal. I look up to him and admire his ability to take care of his family and do every task conscientiously and diligently. My little bro, I'm proud of you as well!

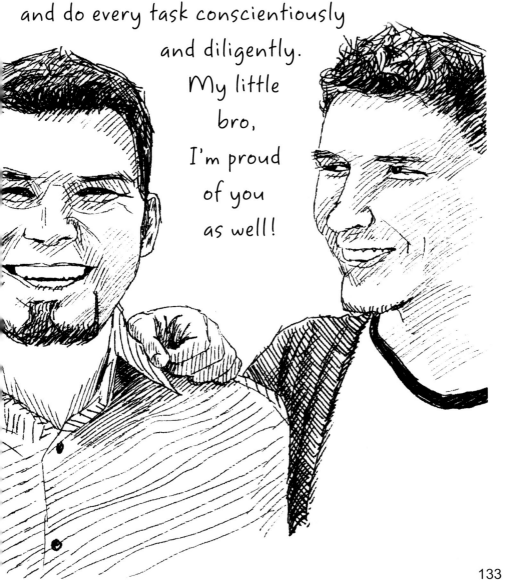

Cancer has a strong grip, not just on the body, but also on the mind. Even though I am "healthy," have not had to face it head-on in a while, it still rears its ugly head. This helps:

"So we're not giving up. How could we! Even though on the outside it often looks like things are falling apart on us, on the inside, where God is making new life, not a day goes by without his unfolding grace."

   – 2 Corinthians 4:16-17 (MSG)

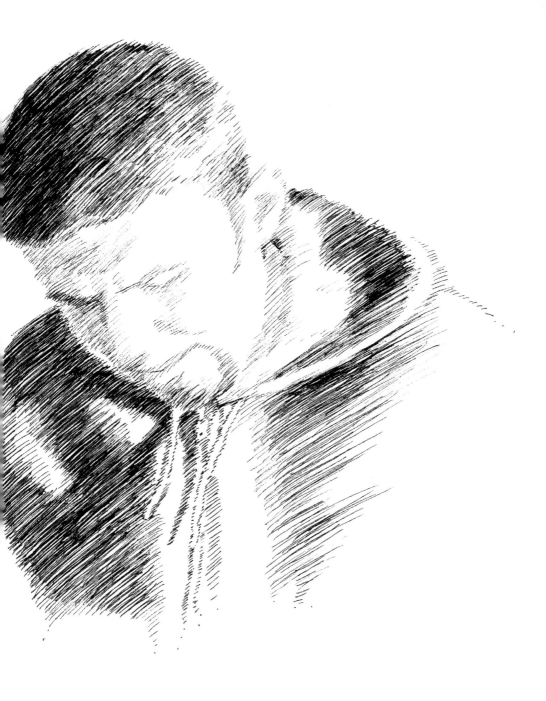

My heart is full, achingly so.
Potential and poison, life and loss,
The moment speaks to me
As I sit listening.

Waves splash ashore; I anticipate
Another moment
Another fullness again ...

This fragile moment is not held
In my arms; I would
Squeeze it too hard.

Instead it is like a breath;
My body craves it
Yet cannot contain it.

This fragile moment is my life
Held by the Creator,
The one who knows the deep,
The one who fills ... continually.

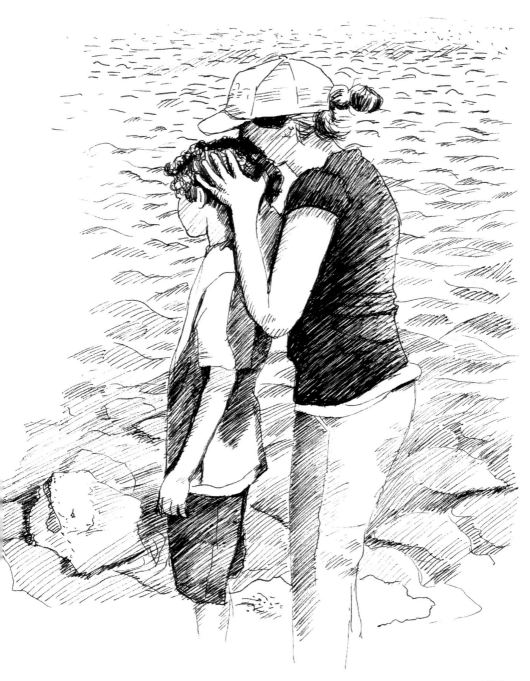

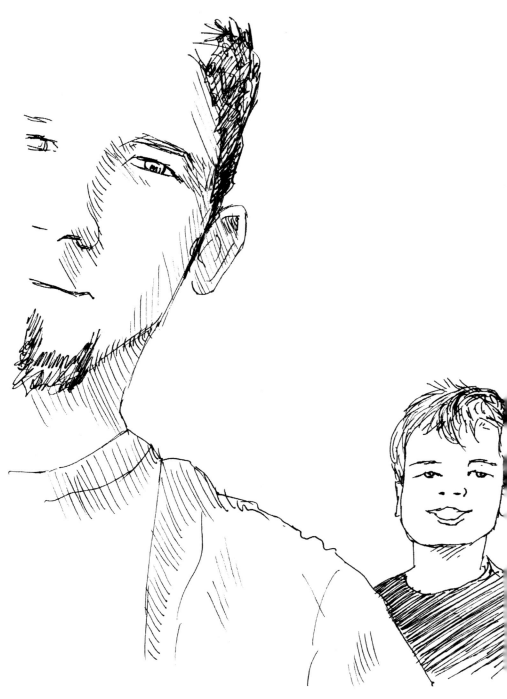

April 2013

In preparation for an upcoming show at the
Bemis Arts building in downtown Seattle,
I work with increased focus on my art. I
can't help but smile at the path my life is
taking, from the chaos of cancer to this
calm felt deep inside when creating images
of my family.

There are still plenty of stressors: money
is tight, work as a teacher never slows
down, and my creative surge could actually
distance me some from my wife and family
as it craves time to explore ideas and to
practice.

Prayer is always a necessity; it is another
word for "balance."

When we are broken and thrown about, our God takes us — right where we are — and shapes us into His artwork.

When we follow Him and obey Him, we become so much more than we could have imagined.

This is why I have come to love the art form of collage. I can bring torn, ripped, fractured, uneven, and discarded papers into a cohesive mix that speaks to a greater truth.

That is what God has done for me. This is my story, and my way of sharing it is through collage.

The materials I use for collage are rather simple, but they give me enormous pleasure:

    a pair of scissors
    some brushes
    a jar of acrylic gel medium.

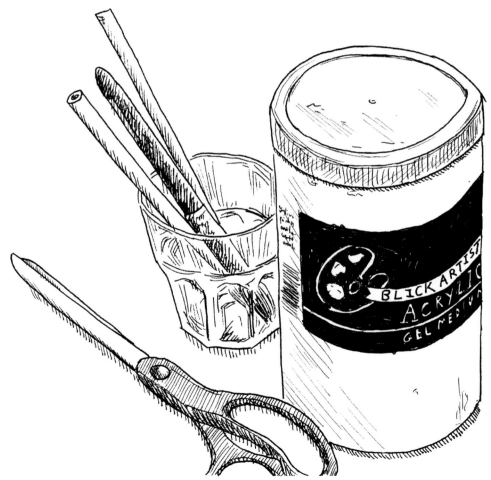

My friend Jimmy Skeen, a pastor, encourages me to share my story during a Sunday service. At first this seems a nice idea, but the thought of sharing my deeply personal experience, for a full hour, to a large crowd, fills me with anxiety.

We plan a more creative approach instead. I will take illustrations and words off the pages of a sketchbook and bring them to life — use visual art to tell a story and give glory to God.

Jimmy patiently instills confidence and provides the support needed.

Instead of using a microphone to speak, I stand on the platform with an easel where I create a "live" collage. Friends come forward to read portions of my story that I have prepared in four

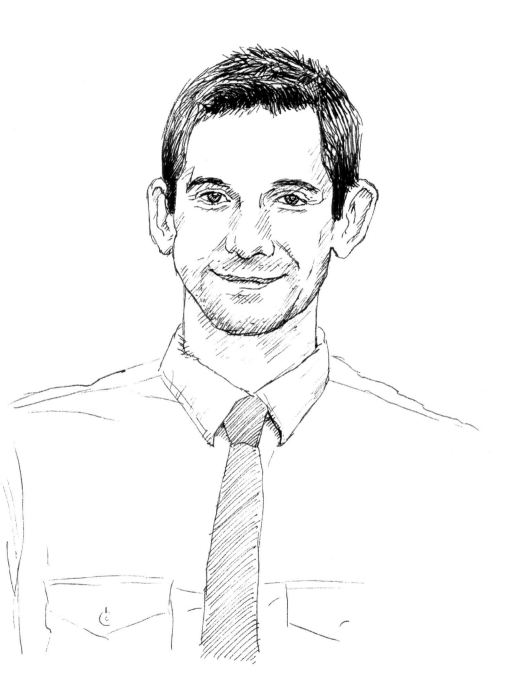

143

separate letters. Each friend also brings some material for me to add to the collage. <u>First</u> come the cancer brochures and papers, which form the dirt (stained brown in advance). <u>Second</u> come maps, which form the roots and sky (the analogy of journey works well). <u>Third</u> come children's picture book covers (leaves), and finally, significant Bible verses (which blend in with the sky).

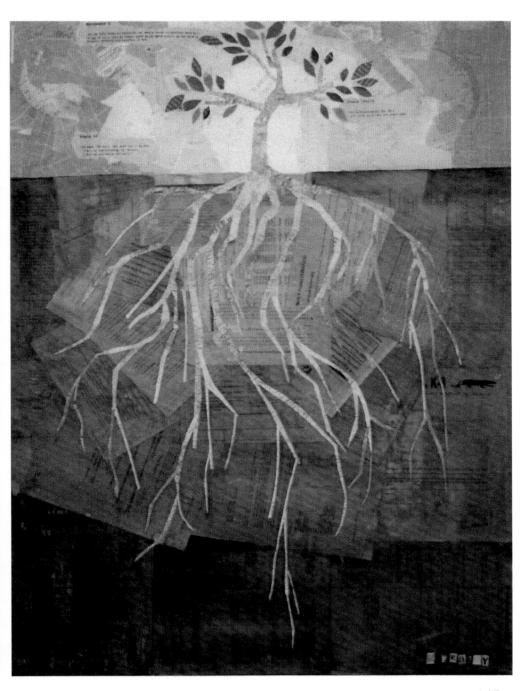

There were moments during my treatment in the spring of 2010 that I felt an absolute peace and calm. All my circumstances were difficult — I felt like crap, looked like crap, couldn't sleep, couldn't focus for more than 5 minutes at a time, had financial strains, etc. Regardless of all this, those moments of peace and calm would carry me over to the next day, next week, or next month. It's hard to describe in words, and I don't have to. Instead, I can speak through my art.

The collages on the following pages were created using children's picture book jackets (the integrity of the book itself was not harmed in the process).

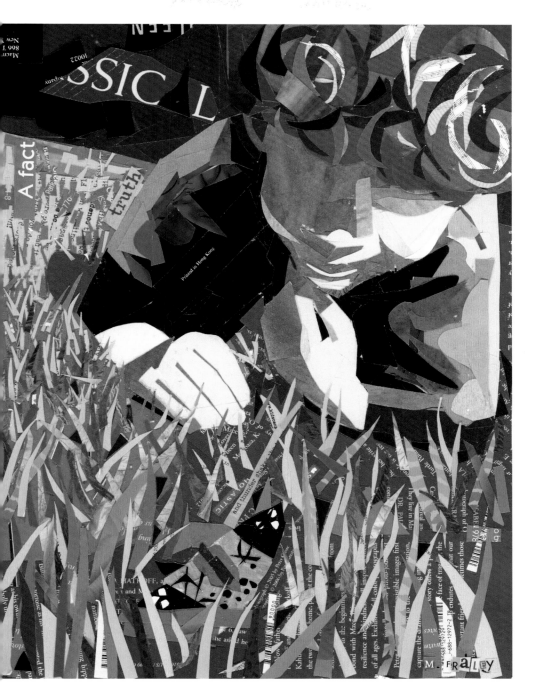

FRONT YARD DISCOVERY

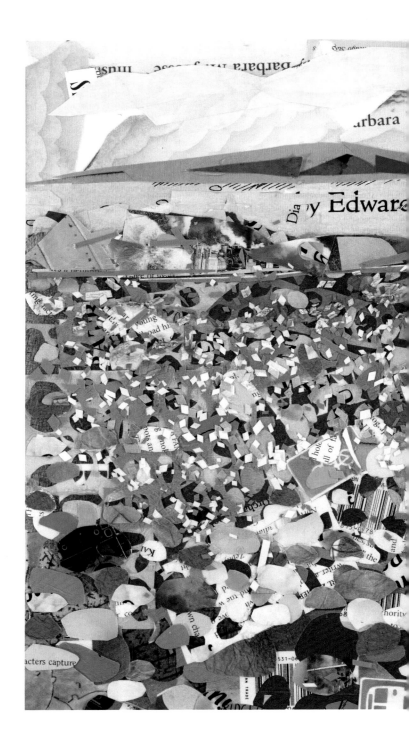

CAMANO BEACH

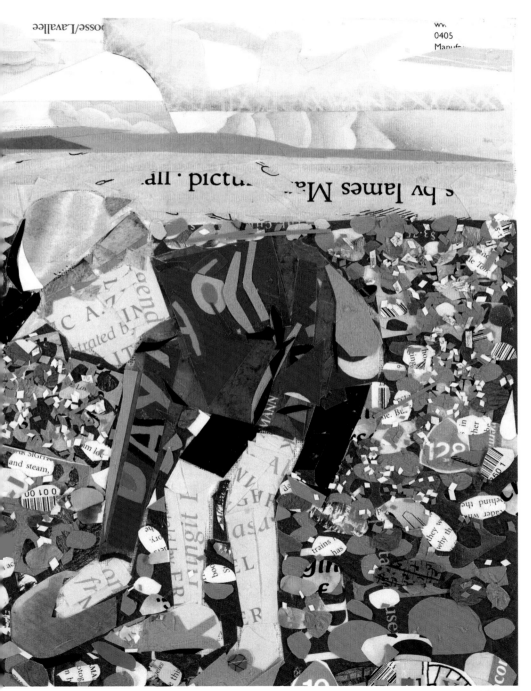

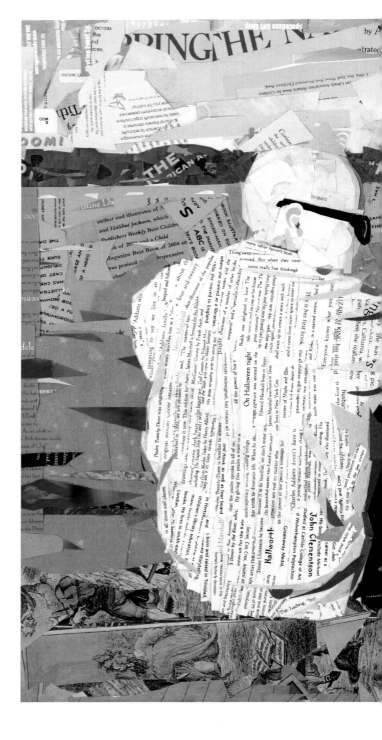

MATTHEW'S BEACH

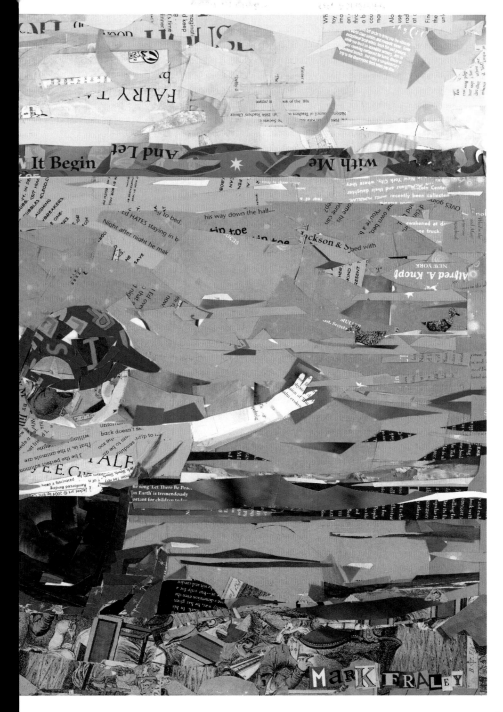

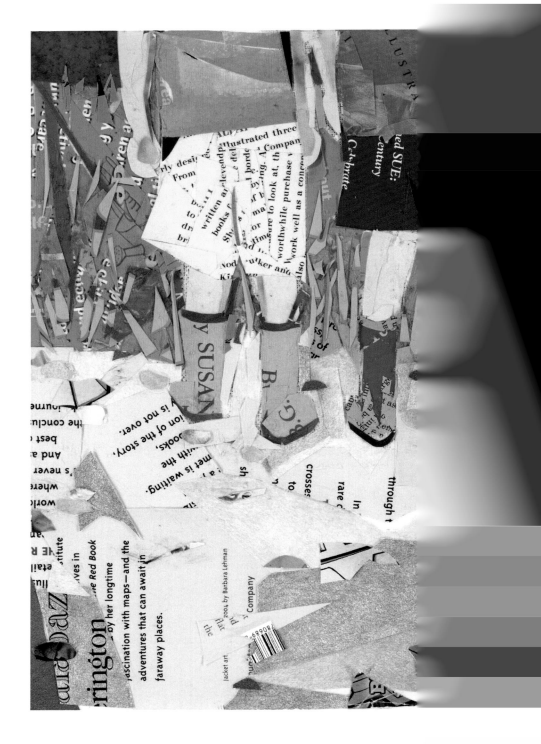

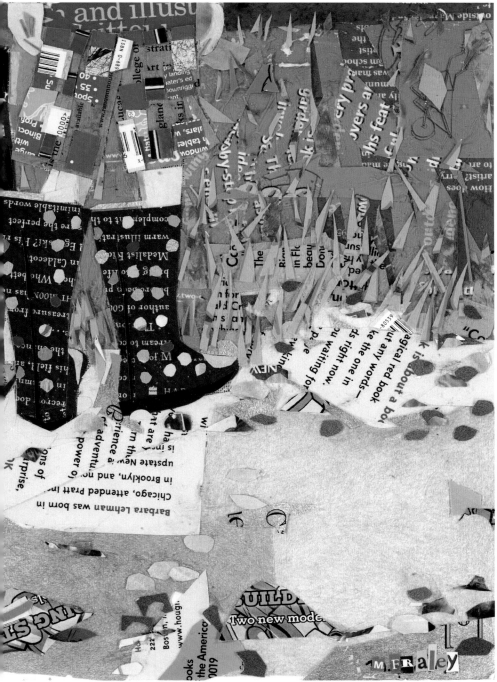

Barbara Lehman was born in Chicago, attended Pratt Institute in Brooklyn, and now lives in upstate New York.

M. Fraley

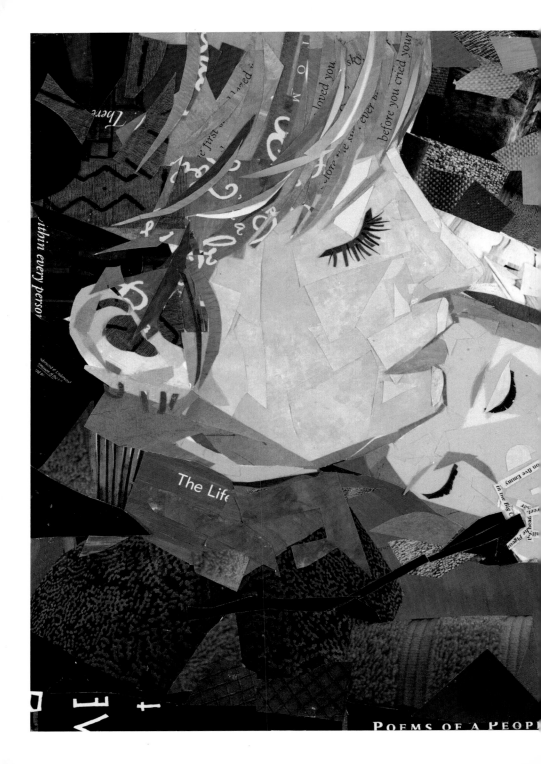

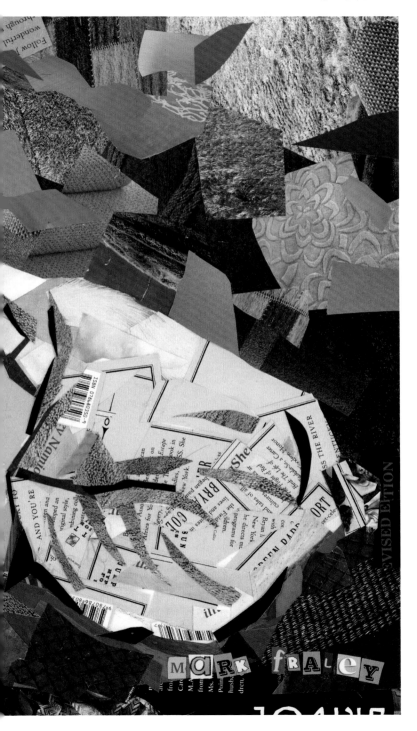

DANS LES BRAS DE MAMAN

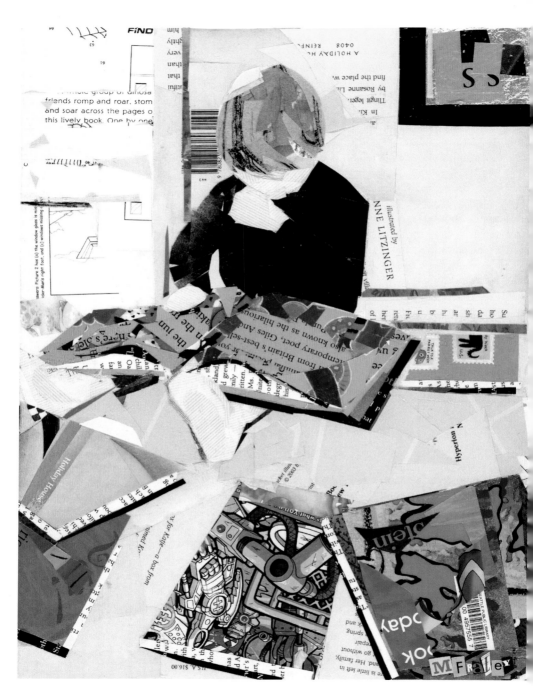

A GOOD READ

AFTERWORD

Every entry in <u>Creation of Calm</u> can be traced back to one of my sketchbooks from the past six years. It may have been a thought written down, an idea scribbled in the corner of a page, a little sketch of my family across a two-page spread … I began using sketchbooks seriously in December of 2007, as I wanted to develop ideas for future paintings and practice my hand at making more realistic portraits. Never did I imagine the shape it would take. Nor did I ever imagine I would be dealing with cancer as a father of young children, just entering my third decade!

The idea of compiling sketchbook entries into a story came when I opened up to others about my battle with cancer. The pages of a sketchbook can be private, and that was how I wanted to keep them. That was my comfort zone. I had control over it and could keep sketching away on my own. But a quiet and insistent voice, that spoke of reaching out and looking to inspire others, pushed me forward.

I was first influenced in sketchbooks through the work of Danny Gregory. In December of 2008, I received as a gift the book <u>An Illustrated Life: Drawing Inspiration from the Private Sketchbooks of Artists, Illustrators, and Designers</u> (2008, F&W Pub). This book opened me up to the many possibilities and shapes a sketchbook could become. I looked up many of the artists that were featured and still follow some of them to this day, notably Cathy Johnson and her Artist Journal Workshop page on Facebook.

My influences span a wide range of artistic domains as long as they contain a heavy dose of creative insight (music, movies, architecture, fashion design, etc.). Often these influences have appeared or become known to me at a critical period in the development of this sketchbook story, Creation of Calm. For instance, I was on my way to work one day, riding the bus and really struggling with finding proper wording to a certain number of sketches I thought were good but simply not connecting when it came to running a narrative next to them. I was listening to NPR, and they were interviewing a poet by the name of Christian Wiman. I had never heard of him before. (In fact, I could only name poets who were probably long deceased.) Christian, who had been fighting cancer bravely for a number of years, was reading excerpts from a recent book release of his poetry, titled Every Riven Thing.

Within just a few uttered lines, I felt the incredible pull of his verse that carried me alongside his experience, and I felt a depth and richness of understanding that could only have been Spirit-led. His description of struggle, but with an element of faith and hope, paralleled what I was trying to say; but it did so with such clarity and outright beauty. After listening to this radio interview, the writing of my own words became much more inspired and life-like.

The Creation of Calm is a continuing story. There is no ending planned, at least not one that I would choose on my own. I want to carry with me all of my experience and use it both for my own growth and for the benefit of others.

I pray that those who view my art and read my story will take a moment to slow down, maybe get off the phone, and just look intently at the everyday they may have overlooked.

For those interested in starting a sketchbook and recording life this way, I have just a few words of encouragement. First, you don't have to set yourself any goal for how your art or your content should develop. It just needs to be honest and straightforward. I had no plan to publish my pages; it still surprises me to this day!

Secondly, find a time each day to put something in your sketchbook. It does not have to be much, you can even tape or glue or put a sticky note of some kind to record a thought, feeling, or event.

Third, find other people who do this activity as well, and build your skill through careful observation. (It is hard not to compare what we do with the work of others. I have other artists who I wish I could emulate better, but that path of comparison leads to stagnation.) Remember: something every day.

And finally — probably the most rewarding aspect of keeping a sketchbook — go back through previous pages you have filled and see the ground you have covered with the help of a loving God. Here is a look at some of my original sketchbook entries:

• An entry from one of my pocket-sized sketchbooks. I distinctly remember a brief moment of clarity I had to write down these words. I did not have a picture in mind for these specific words other than a cartoonish version of myself waiting for something, maybe at the doctor's office.

• A self-portrait practice, one that I made with no specific goal in mind other than capturing a feeling or expression. After completing it and letting it sit in my sketchbook for a while, I returned to it and realized this drawing paired well with the statement about "there's a sadness that exists…"

Pages of my sketchbooks talk to each other; and when I read back over them, I often find ideas that can be developed further. And when I look back through my pages, I often just say, "Thank you, Jesus."

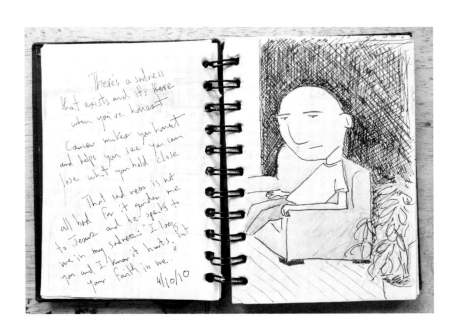

There's a sadness
that exists and it's there
when you've honest.
Cancer makes you honest
and helps you see you can
lose what you hold close

That sadness is but
all bad for it guides me
to Jesus and he sparks to
me in my sadness..." I love
you and I know it hurts, but
your faith in me."
4/10/10

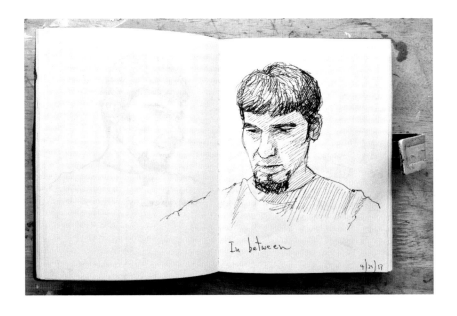

In between
4/25/18

My favorite Bible verses for creative inspiration:

"Behold, This Dreamer cometh..." (Genesis 37:19, KJV). I like the idea that a dreamer can be dangerous.

"Be imitators of God therefore, as dearly beloved children" (Ephesians 5:1, ISV). I see this verse as an invitation to be creative.

"Make a careful exploration of who you are and the work you have been given, and then sink yourself into that. Don't be impressed with yourself. Don't compare yourself to others. Each of us must take responsibility for doing the creative best you can with your own life" (Galatians 6:4-5, MSG).

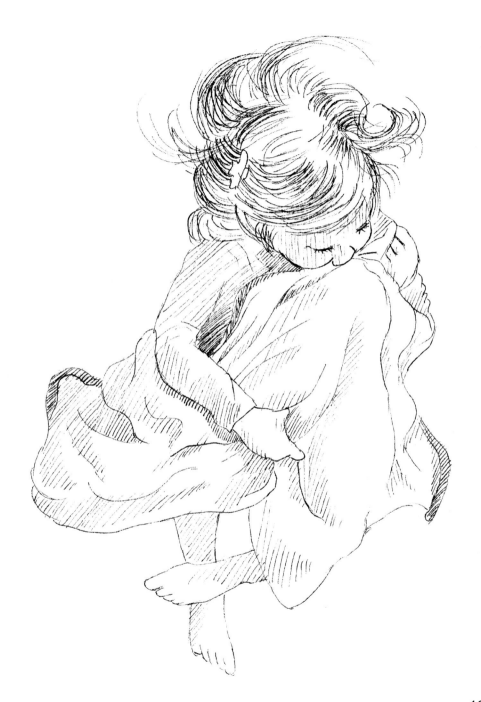

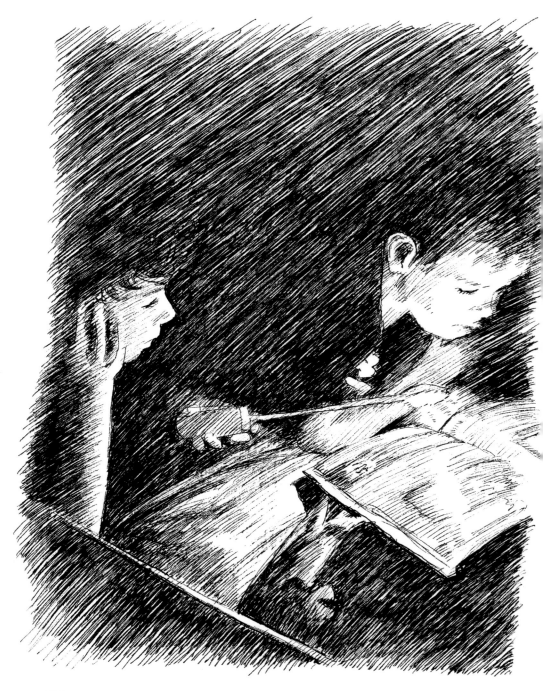

CONCLUSION

I continue to find inspiration in everyday life. These little moments, when gathered together, create a narrative of hope.

With all that can go wrong and seems messed up in the world, these few moments can appear as gifts and speak to the greater truth that requires a little reflection and patience to find.

April 2014

On our way to Easter
Sunday service.

We now live in Colorado;
we have a new home,
a new church, a new
school for the kids, new
jobs, and many other new
things that can easily
turn into worries.

What's next is a question
full of promise, provided I
keep my focus and "calm."

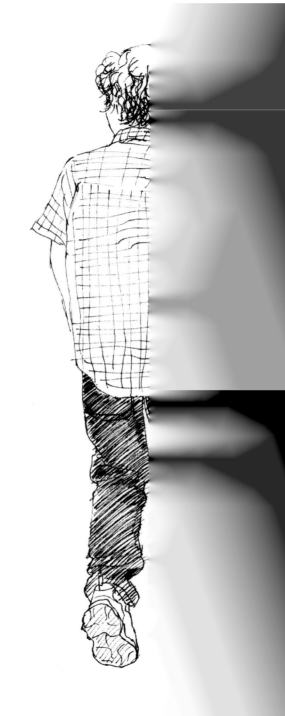

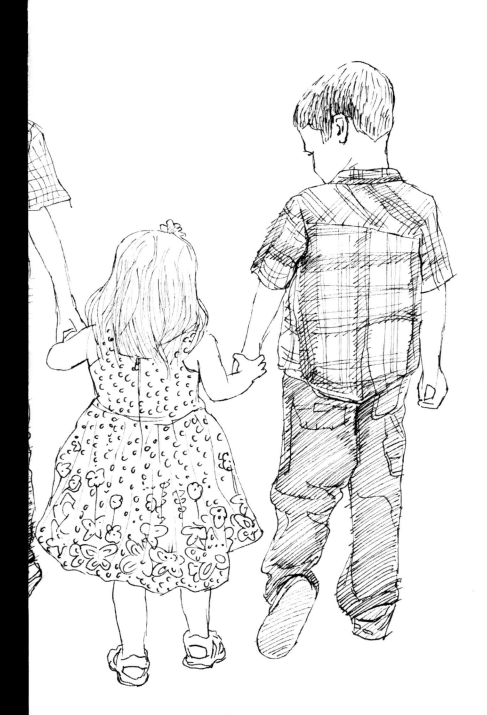

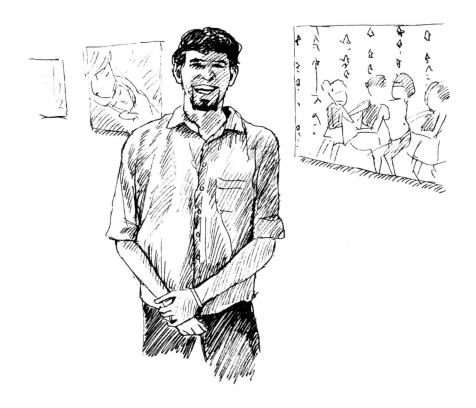

About the Author/Artist

Mark Fraley grew up in France as a child of Christian missionaries. From a young age, he drew countless pictures, including cars, jets, and dogs. This passion for putting pen to paper came into full bloom when faced with the challenge of his life, cancer. His family—his three kids and his wife—brought the calm needed to face this battle with courage, and God placed a deep-rooted peace that remained beyond just the moment of fervent prayer. He works as an early-childhood educator in Colorado.

To follow Mark on Facebook, visit Mark Fraley Art. To view more of his collages and artwork, visit www.markfraleyart.com.